D1349340

Fundamentals of
MEDICAL
MANAGEMENT

A Guide for the New Physician Executive

Edited by Jerry L. Hammon, MD, FACPE

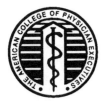

The American College of Physician Executives
Two Urban Centre, Suite 200
4890 West Kennedy Boulevard
Tampa, Florida 33609-2575
813/287-2000

Copyright ©1993 by the American College of Physician Executives.
Reproduction or translation of this work beyond that permitted by copyright
law without permission of the College is prohibited. Requests for permission to
reprint or for further information should be directed to ACPE, Two Urban
Centre, Suite 200, 4890 West Kennedy Boulevard, Tampa, Florida 33609-2575.

ISBN: 0-924674-17-2

Library of Congress Card Number: 92-72278

Printed in the United States of America by Lithocolor, Tampa, Florida.

PREFACE

✦

*F*or several years now, the American College of Physician Executives has conducted a group of special educational programs intended for physicians who are just entering the first stages of medical management. Aimed at medical staff leaders and at department and section chiefs, these courses introduce the fundamentals of management to help these individuals understand the nature of the task that they have undertaken. These courses are different from the College's Physician in Management seminar series, in that they provide only a few critical survival skills. They are not intended to build a solid foundation in management.

Many of the graduates of these courses have indicated both an interest in and a need for a reference that would remind them of the content of courses after they return to their organizations. And so this new book from the College have been developed. Members of the College's Society on Hospitals took undertook the project, many of them serving as authors of chapters. Dr. Jerry Hammon, the editor, was Chair of the Society during the book project and volunteered to oversee its design and production. He has carefully read every manuscript, offering guidance for revisions as necessary. His foreword tells much about the intent and design of the publication.

Combined with *New Leadership in Health Care Management: The Physician Executive*, another hardcover book in the College's catalog of publications, this new offering not only assists the physician new to medical management to deal effectively with his or her new responsibilities but also further defines and refines the medical management profession itself. There are all manner of environments and levels of responsibility in the medical management profession. *Fundamentals of Medical Management: A Guide for the New Physician Executive* is where it all begins.

Roger Schenke
American College of Physician Executives
Tampa, Florida
January 4, 1993

FOREWORD

*L*et's flash back to a summer day many years ago, when my friend Don said to me, "Let's go swimming in the river."

My answer was, "I'm afraid to, because I've never been in deep water and I don't know how to swim."

Don insisted, "Come along, and I'll help you learn to swim. I'll also show you how to avoid some of those deadly currents that could even cause a good swimmer to be eliminated."

Reluctantly, I answered, "Okay, but I'm still a bit concerned that I won't like it well enough to spend the time learning to be a good enough swimmer to survive in really fast, deep water."

As usual, Don said, "Don't worry. We won't get into that kind of trouble if we just stay in the shallow back water where we know we can stand up and really concentrate on learning to be strong swimmers. Then we can venture out into the deeper water with the treacherous currents. You will feel very much at home in deep, swift water by that time."

Let us look at a similar flashback to some 15 years ago, when I was first asked to become a full-time administrator in a large hospital. The offer was for me to temporarily fill this position, for three or four months. My answer was very similar to the answer about going swimming in deep water. "I don't know anything about being an administrator of a hospital, especially a big one, and I'm afraid of getting in over my head." My friend gently urged me to take the position. He assured me that from his position as administrative assistant, plus with help from a very excellent executive secretary, I could fulfill the duties of administrator. He also suggested that I could even become confident enough to want to explore administration as a new career.

In both instances, I listened and I learned. Today, I am a very strong swimmer. I have also been complimented for being a competent medical executive. Neither would have been possible without the patient tutoring and support of my friends.

My early pursuit of a permanent, full-time career as a physician executive was greatly enhanced by becoming a member of the American Academy of Medical Directors, now known as the American College of Physician Executives and also by enrolling in the first of the "Physician in Management" seminars sponsored by the organization. But the years prior to the PIM courses would have been much easier and more meaningful had I had access to a "handy little manual" for medical managers. This monograph is just such a manual. It is intended to keep you afloat while you learn how to navigate all the swift and deep waters of medical management. Each of the chapters will assist you in solving problems associated with managing physicians, administrators, and your time.

Confidence in mastering the many facets of administration will, I'm sure, pique your interest in diving into a larger administrative position. Remember, this handy little monograph has been written by professionals who also got their starts by learning to swim in the safer, shallow waters of management before progressing to the major waters for physician executives.

Good luck!

Jerry L. Hammon, MD, FACPE
West Milton, Ohio
January 4, 1993

TABLE OF CONTENTS

Table of Contents

CHAPTER 1

Life as a Medical Manager

by Laurence G. Roth, MD

What does it mean to be a medical director, a vice president for medical affairs, or a physician executive with a related title that says you are involved in the business side of medicine? Within every group of physicians or other health care providers large enough to require leadership and management, there is a potential position for a physician executive. Opportunities are found in group practices, hospital and medical staff administration, larger institutions providing managed care at multiple sites, and in sections within these organizations. There are medical managers in industries producing equipment, supplies, and pharmaceuticals; in research programs; and in the many agencies of local, state, and federal government. In recognition of the need for medical management, the military has been sending its personnel for training and experience so that they can qualify for assignments with managerial responsibilities. There is also increasing awareness of the appropriateness of medical management in academia.

Although the titles of these positions vary widely (chief executive officer, chief operations officer, chief medical officer, vice president of medical affairs, medical director, department chief, section chief, and many more), all of them involve managing people and programs, as contrasted with treating patients in clinical specialties. Managers also attend meetings and handle a lot of paperwork. Of course, there is some of both of these activities in clinical practice, but there are more meetings and much more paperwork for managers. Managing people, however, is the keystone of management. This chapter is an introduction to the general aspects of medical management as the profession is now constituted and an indication of its future possibilities.

There is no way of predicting how widespread the requirement may become in the United States, but when New York State revised its hospital code in 1988,[1] it included a simple statement that firmly established medical management at every hospital in the state. The code says that the "governing board shall appoint a physician, referred to as the medical director, who shall be responsible for directing the medical staff organization." This action in New York may well foreshadow coming events in other states. A conclusion now being reached in New York is that medical directors are doing things that had not been done previously, and hospitals would no longer be willing to do without them because the benefits have been significant. Another conclusion is that the role of medical management is not for a casual participant. It is an important function best served by those who have the essential qualifications to be medical managers.

The New York State definition of the position's responsibility establishes the hospital medical director as the focus of attention in medical matters for the medical staff, administration, and the governing board. The definition serves as a useful beginning for understanding what it means to be a medical director or a physician executive generally. It emphasizes the interesting and challenging role that the medical director assumes in being the advocate for each one of the three entities to the other two in a hospital environment, but the medical manager role is similar regardless of the environment in which the person serves.

The liaison and advocacy role of the medical director is essential in any operation where successfully getting and giving information on medical matters is of paramount importance. For example, the medical manager's role in quality assurance and risk management will demand constant emphasis on adequate communication and documentation. In this, as in other aspects of medical management, the medical director should expect to set an example of how to communicate with everyone and how to properly document findings, recommendations, and actions.

In the transition from clinical practice to medical management, most of the characteristics of clinician must give way to those of the manager, but there is one feature of clinical practice that is retained in the transition without loss of significance. It is most important for the medical manager to continue to be an advocate for the patient. In evaluating medical care and reviewing medical staff practices, there is a unique opportunity for the medical manager to facilitate achievement of what is best for the patient. Other actors in the organization may have concerns about cost containment or avoidance of liability and personal preferences that affect their actions and their subsequent decisions. A medical manager is usually not encumbered to the same degree by these considerations and can speak to what is in the best interests of the patient.

Planning products, services, and programs and devising innovations to make improvements in an organization's operations are among the ways in which the medical manager contributes to the successful outcome of the work of the organization. Generally, the activities of the medical manager, especially in a provider setting, are still tied, even if indirectly, to health care delivery. Modern medical management, for instance, gives increasing attention to what is termed "continuous quality improvement" or "total quality management." These new medical quality management approaches represent adaptations of principles established in industry that are proving to be of great value in health care.[2-4] (Medical quality management concepts are discussed in detail in Chapter 12 of this book.) Crosby[5] has written about the concept, "Do it right the first time." That is a goal for every patient-physician encounter, and a great guideline for every medical manager.

In order to play a leading role in the design and implementation of programs that address medical quality and other issues of current concern, the medical manager must learn a wide variety of new and very different concepts and skills. The learning that must take place is especially intense for the newly recruited medical manager who is just beginning to gain experience.

The manager is an important support person. Vested with central responsibility and authority, the medical manager works with and for many people who come for advice and direction. The manager assists others in carrying out tasks that they might not otherwise be able to accomplish. The medical manager helps others to overcome their reluctance to follow through on programs and projects and helps them avoid or overcome obstacles to progress.

The medical manager operates out of what becomes a central command post. Information comes from administration, the governing board, and the medical staff and its committees. With knowledge of the resources available and of what has to be done, the position becomes akin to the President's Chief of Staff in relation to the leaders of the U.S. Senate and House of Representatives. There is the need and the opportunity to assist in devising policy and then seeing that it is carried out, all the while being responsible to those whom she or he serves. The guidance of the medical manager is especially important for members of the medical staff who have leadership responsibilities but who perhaps lack the knowledge, motivation, or time to carry out those responsibilities.

A manager also serves as a counselor to the many individuals who come to be listened to, to be encouraged, and to be guided to solutions they find acceptable. The availability of the medical manager leads to the solution of many problems that might otherwise persist and cause trouble. Existence of the position is a signal to practitioners and others that help is available from a person who understands their concerns.

There is a significant relationship between the medical manager and new members of the medical staff. The indoctrination that is essential starts each physician off in harmony with the way things are done locally. This opens communication that can be used in other matters. There are always problems for the new physician with the various regulatory agencies, and guidance here can eliminate a lot of grief later. If the medical manage has an effective open door policy, physicians feel free to come in and discuss potential as well as real problems that pertain to them as individuals or to their relationships with committees and departments. Many of these encounters are unscheduled. The medical manager's just being available is most helpful to everyone concerned.

In a recent report about hospital-based physician executives based on a 12-year, ongoing study, Lloyd and Guilfoyle describe the medical manager as follows: "The profile that emerges is a 53 year-old white male, working almost 50 hours a week in a full-time position, appointed by the hospital and reporting to the chief executive officer. This individual is board certified and has major responsibilities for quality assurance, credentialing, risk management, and utilization review. His or her salary is into six figures."[6] The report provides other details that relate to the varieties of opportunities for medical managers. It should be reviewed by anyone who is seriously considering such a career. Because of the duration of this continuing study and the many different components of the study, this is probably the most valuable resource for anyone who is seriously considering the switch to medical management.

The medical manager has a position of influence. This influence is derived to a large extent from the organizational authority necessary to be an effective leader with major responsibilities. But it is also a result of the manager's effectiveness in processing information, such as external regulations and internal policies that affect the personnel and the work of the organization. Interpretation and application of these regulations and policies are an important part of the medical manager's job and have a significant impact on the operation of the organization. The busy practitioner does not have time to investigate all of the information that is available. By attending meetings at which in-depth discussions are conducted and having time to read materials that are circulated, the medical manager becomes a resource that permits pragmatic application of this information through reliable advice.

The opportunity to be the one to receive information and to give advice allows the medical manager to greatly affect the smoothness of the organization's work and the satisfaction of everyone's work life. The medical manager accomplishes much of this in the role of an educator, both directly and indirectly. In many situations, it is the medical manager who is in charge of continuing education programs. The medical staff is consulted as to its special needs, programs are arranged locally when feasible, and other sources of education are developed. The medical manager is also an educator by example and through counseling of both individuals and groups with whom he or she comes in contact.

The medical manager faces the paradox of being an advocate for "good," as in responsibilities for medical quality management, while also being a target for criticism when perceived to be the source of something "bad," as in dealing with inappropriate or disruptive physician behavior and its associated problems. The former achievements will often be taken for granted by the organization and the latter will consume both time and energy with little in the way of positive recognition. Self-confidence and the ability to evaluate performance objectively are essential in both cases. The ultimate achievement for the manager is self-management, dealing with the responsibilities that are part of the management package with fairness and forthrightness. The manager is a large, visible target for anyone with an axe to grind and is infrequently rewarded with praise. The job requires a well-honed ability to cope with these facts of management life.

Management skills are not an inherent part of any person's abilities. They have to be acquired. As they are used and mistakes are made, the skills become increasingly effective. But the necessary skills have to be actively identified and then aggressively sought and polished. A major purpose of the American College of Physician Executives is to provide opportunities for management education.[7] Its goal is to introduce physicians interested in pursuing a management career to the full range of knowledge and skills that they will need for success. Of course, an allied purpose is to provide these educational opportunities in a setting and at a pace that is least disruptive to physicians' professional and personal lives. For some, however, programs leading to master's level degrees are possible and preferable. Several opportunities for master's degrees specifically oriented to medical management have recently been developed and others are certain to follow. Significantly, the American Board of Medical Management now identifies those who have reached a level of knowledge and experience that qualifies them to be certified as Diplomates in medical management.

The field of medical management is growing rapidly, so there will be many future opportunities, both for those already in the profession and for those who have just begun an investigation of the alternative. It is always a good idea to talk with someone who is a practicing medical manager and to learn how that person came to be in that position. The educational programs and conferences of the American College of Physician Executives are excellent experiences that allow exploration of the career of medical management. They are also an opportunity to meet many individuals with similar interests and varying degrees of experience.

The management career will not have universal appeal for physicians. But for those who are interested, the opportunities are good and the work is satisfying. This book is intended to help practicing physicians with some curiosity about such a career to determine if it fits their needs and to help them understand the road that will have to be traveled to achieve success.

References

1. New York State Public Health Law Part 405, Subchapter A of Chapter V, Title 10, Sections 405.2 (e) (2), and 405.4.

2. Scherkenbach, W. *The Deming Route to Quality and Productivity: Road Maps and Road Blocks*. Washington, D.C.: George Washington University, Cee Press Books, 1988.

3. Juran, J. *Juran on Planning for Quality*. New York, N.Y.: Free Press, 1988.

4. Berwick, D., and others. *Curing Health Care—New Strategies for Quality Improvement*. San Francisco, Calif.: Jossey-Bass Publishers, 1990.

5. Crosby, P. *Quality without Tears: The Art of Hassle-Free Management.* New York, N.Y.: McGraw Hill, 1984.

6. Lloyd, J., and Guilfoyle, F. "Physician Executives in the '90s: Report of a National Survey. *Physician Executive* 17(2):23-9, March-April 1991.

7. *New Leadership in Health Care Management: The Physician Executive.* Curry, W., Ed., Tampa, Fla.: American College of Physician Executives, 1988.

Laurence G. Roth, MD, is Medical Director, Genesee Memorial Hospital, Batavia, New York.

CHAPTER 2

Organization Theory

by Robert Inguagiato, MBA

*F*or a health care professional who is relatively new to the role of organizational manager, the dynamics of organizations can be exhilarating, challenging, confusing, and sometimes contradictory. For many physicians who have been nonmanagerial participants in organizations, the organization was a means to an end—a place to practice professional competency. In management, the focus shifts to creating and managing the organization where professional competencies are practiced. Your training, skills, and talents were crucial precursors to your entering the managerial world. But you will quickly find out that your new role requires something more of you. You will need managerial and leadership competencies, in addition to the competencies you have been rewarded for in the past.

The pursuit of these managerial and leadership competencies can seem disparate. Organizational, leadership, and managerial theories abound in today's literature. Which ones should you choose, which ones should you believe, and which ones are accurate? The answer is all of them and none of them. You should choose the ones that will allow you to add value to your constituencies: patients, staff, CEO, board, and community at large.

Organization theory places meaning and understanding on the dynamics operating in organizations. You will find it helpful to have one, if not several, paradigms available to interpret the forces at play in organizations. My bias is to provide you with a simple model that explains many of the complexities of organization life, rather than a complex model that explains the simplicities of organization life.

This chapter has four objectives:

✦ To explain the three phases of organizational growth.

✦ To discuss the behavioral characteristics of these three phases.

✦ To take an exploratory look at the variables that create the dynamic ebb and flow of organization life.

✦ To put this all together through the eyes of the manager

The Three Phases of Organizational Growth

Most organizations will undergo three distinct phases of evolution or growth that will often be characterized by how the organization is structured. These growth phases can be observed at the macro level (the entire organization), or they may be seen at the micro level (a department). Often, the way a department is structured will be characteristic of the developmental phase of the entire organization. Observing the structure of an organization will tell you much about how decisions are made, the level of trust, the level of maturity, the management styles that are likely to prevail, and the behavioral expectations placed on staff.

"Dependency" is the first phase of organizational growth. Organizational structures that produce highly dependent behavior in their staffs can be characterized as being very young in their developmental growth. Dependent organizations can be old in years but young in their development. Conversely, organizations that are young in years may be more developed in their growth cycle, and this will be evidenced by their organizational structure. A dependent organization is analogous to a child who is dependent upon parents for most major life-support systems. Decision making is highly centralized. At times, this will be characterized by a large headquarters staff. The working environment is highly control-oriented, and decision making is in the hands of a relative few. This dependency phase can be seen in start-up ventures where experience and maturity are low, or in departments that are either new or in trouble. The level of trust in highly dependent organizations is low. People are expected to do as they are told, and behaviors that cause waves are quickly extinguished. This type of organization generally rewards autocratic leadership behavior for those who are among the chosen few. It is rare to see participative management styles used with any success in a department or organization of this nature.

The second phase is "Independence." It is common to have an organization grow from a highly dependent structure to one of independence. This phase of organizational growth is analogous to a young adult who strikes off on his or her own. On an organizational level, this independence would be characterized by departments' and functions' being highly independent of each other. Each would make decisions with its own immediate world in mind. This form of organization structure is more evolved than the dependent form discussed previously. Decision making is decentralized, departments and functions operate in an autonomous manner, and individual performance is highly cherished. There is little emphasis placed on interdepartmental relationships, and at times staff will wonder if they are all working for the same institution. This type of organizational structure can breed a high level of internal competition that, if not carefully monitored, can cause counterproductive outcomes. The level of trust in an independent organization is generally high, and the level of control, evidenced by organizational systems, is considerably lower than in a dependent organization. An independent organization is more mature and expresses confidence in its staff members' abilities.

The first two phases of organizational growth, dependency and independence, are the ruling majority in health care organizations and can be successful under the right conditions. However, each has a major drawback. The dependent organization does not fully utilize the talents of its staff members and runs the risk of not treating them with dignity. The independent organization uses and recognizes the talents of individual staff members but often loses the synergy available through cross-functional cooperation and collaboration.

A third phase of growth has been developing over the past decade. Interdependence characterizes this third phase of growth. An interdependent organization takes the best of the dependent and independent structures and adds one additional element—synergy. An interdependent organization or department would have a decentralized decision-making process; however, there would be a strong emphasis on not making decisions in a vacuum. Departments would be encouraged, if not required, to consult with other areas of the institution to discuss the ramifications of decisions, and in most cases a collaborative approach would be emphasized. At the department level, a strong emphasis would be placed on the need for professionals from different areas or backgrounds to come together in the decision-making process. Again, the collaborative approach would be evident in the day-to-day life of the department. There is a strong emphasis placed on interdepartmental cooperation rather than interdepartmental competition. Although individual contributors are considered important, there is a higher value placed on teamwork. The synergy of cross-functional cooperation and collaboration is an expected outcome of organizations or departments that have an interdependent structure.

Behavioral Characteristics of Growth Phases

Why is it necessary to identify the key behavioral characteristics for these developmental phases? The answer is congruency. If you expect the staff in your department or organization to behave in certain ways, you must have an understanding of what behaviors your organizational structure is shaping and reinforcing. For example, it is particularly frustrating for a manager to expect his or her staff to exhibit collaborative behaviors when the departmental structure is causing and reinforcing people to behave independently of each other. As a manager, if there is congruency among your organizational structure, systems, and managerial behavior, there is a higher likelihood that your staff will behave in ways that will meet your expectations. Naturally, your expectations should be based on realistic outcomes of these forces or you will be disappointed. The following information is designed to help you identify realistic behavioral expectations based on these three organizational growth phases.

A dependent organization produces staff behaviors that are hinged on a very few people providing direction for the entire staff. Consequently, if you expect your staff to be self-directional, a dependent organizational structure will not produce such behaviors. The staff will not have a feeling of empowerment. As a result, you should not expect staff members to take matters into their own hands if a situation calls for action beyond their specific job description. Individual discretionary effort would not be reinforced in a dependent organization.

Dependent organizations tend to produce consistent but rarely superior performance. If you need consistently average performance, a dependent organization may well help you achieve that goal. Dependent organizations produce a low level of innovation. This is particularly true if you expect staff members to be innovators. What innovation is developed must come from the few decision makers in the organization. If the organization has exacting work systems and procedures in place that reduce the need for individual judgment, the level of efficiency in the organization could be high. However, without these systems and procedures in place, the level of efficiency in the organization could be very disappointing. Professional work standards must be articulated in fine detail if you expect the staff to meet these criteria. This is true in a dependent organization where staff are dependent upon the parents of the organization for all their needs. As you have observed, a dependent organization produces and reinforces a host of staff behaviors. What is crucial for you is to be aware of what you are asking for when you develop a Dependent organization. If your managerial expectations are congruent with the outcomes of a dependent organization, you will not be disappointed.

An independent organization produces and reinforces a different set of staff behaviors. Staff members will be encouraged to be more self-directive in their day-to-day work. It is not unusual to have reward systems in an independent organization that reinforce individual initiative. Staff members will often use discretionary effort to accomplish their work. If a situation calls for an individual to do more than his or her job description states, it is not unusual for that individual to go beyond the call of duty. Independent organizations tend to produce a higher level of overall individual performance. However, it is likely that there may be more downward blips on the performance screen as well. Whereas a dependent organization will produce a consistent average performance and very little, if any, superior performance, an independent organization will produce more variability in performance but a higher likelihood of more superior staff performance.

The level of innovation by individual staff members in an independent organization could be high, if the organization's reward system encourages such behavior. The structure of an independent organization would certainly provide the support base for innovation to be part of an individual's behavioral repertoire. The pressure on the organization to provide exacting detail on the professional work standards expected of individuals is considerably lighter than in a dependent organization. The independent organization is very individual-oriented;

thus staff members are encouraged and expected to have their own internal standards of quality, in addition to what may be formally spelled out by the organization. An independent organization places a great deal of emphasis on individual and departmental autonomy, which produces staff behavior that is congruent with this structure and phase of growth. If your expectations as a department manager or chief of staff are congruent with the type of organization you create, the likelihood of your being confused or frustrated by staff behaviors are lessened considerably.

An interdependent organization encourages collaborative and cooperative staff behaviors. As in an independent organization, staff members are likely to express self-direction. However, the interdependent organization will encourage and reinforce self-directive behaviors that take into account other people and other departments, rather than self-directive behavior that is individual-oriented. Staff members will generally behave in ways that reflect a sense of empowerment and also will demonstrate a sense of responsibility for other staff members' work. They not only will perform their jobs but often will go beyond them if the situation calls for more discretion. Staff of an Interdependent organization tend to behave in ways that demonstrate a concern for the global good of the organization, rather than focusing individually.

An interdependent organization, similar to an Independent organization, is likely to produce superior performance. However, this superior performance will be more observable on an organizationwide basis, rather than an individual or department level. The amount of discretionary effort individual staff members may exhibit to accomplish their work can be quite high, especially when they see the ramifications of actions on the entire organization. The level of innovation in an interdependent organization can be even higher than in an independent organization. The synergistic effect of collaboration between individuals and departments stimulates the level of innovation. The organization will not need to spell out in exacting detail individual work standards, but can paint a vision of the expected outcomes of the team. An interdependent organization emphasizes team performance and collaboration rather than individual performance. Individual performance is valued in an interdependent organization. However, relationships and their impact on the overall performance of the organization are valued even more.

Understanding the behavioral characteristics of the different stages of organizational growth will often explain why individuals, departments, and organizations behave the way they do. The main issue is congruency. If your expectations are congruent with the stage of your organization's growth, the likelihood of behavioral outcomes being what you desired are high. Additionally, there are other variables that affect the performance of an organization or department. These variables, in combination with the stage of organizational growth, will have a major impact on the behavioral performance of individuals and, subsequently, the organization.

Dynamic Variables of Organizational Life

The stage of organizational life, i.e., dependent, independent, or interdependent, and its corresponding behavioral characteristics are major contributors to shaping organizational life. However, they are not the only variables at play in this dynamic ebb and flow. There are five other components that help shape life in organizations: espoused organizational values, mission/goals, systems (psychological and technical), external competition, and management behavior.

The espoused values of an organization, and on a micro level of a department, help create behavioral expectations. If a health care organization states that one of its fundamental values is to provide a working environment that encourages individual initiative, it is stating a behavioral expectation that it has of its staff. Concurrently, this value statement is also saying that staff can expect the organization to behave in a manner that will support and encourage this behavior. The adage, "Be careful of what you ask for because you are likely to get it," is a critical factor in organizational values. Organizational values help create the rules of the game for organizational life. If the rules are broken, incongruence develops. Once this occurs it is difficult to understand and shape behavior, and the impact of other variables becomes less predictable.

The mission and goals of the organization help create a sense of purpose and direction that tell staff members what game they are participating in. If a health care organization states that one of its goals is to provide the highest quality of patient care, its staff will use this goal to provide direction for day-to-day behavior. However, if staff members observe the organization continually making exceptions to this goal, they can only interpret this behavior as the new goal. Inevitably, inconsistencies such as this are what create new organizational goals, much to the surprise of the organization.

Organizational systems, both psychological and technical, have a major impact on organizational life. Psychological systems, such as performance appraisals, internal newsletters, compensation plans, career progression systems, and organizational role models, will shape the behavior and performance of staff members in a powerful way. For example, if a health care organization has an espoused value of only hiring the best professionals in the field and a performance appraisal system that forces the majority of appraisees to be evaluated as adequate, staff members will soon get the message that adequate behavior is all that is really wanted in the organization. Inevitably, this outcome will come as a surprise to the organization and to any manager who is on the receiving side of this behavior.

Technical systems, such as management information reports, the budget process, and resource acquisition systems, will have an impact on the life and behavior of staff members as well. For example, if an organization is in its independent stage of growth and has a resource acquisition system that requires

CEO approval for the most insignificant purchases, a staff member will become confused about the message the organization is attempting to deliver.

External competition can have a substantial impact on the stress an organization experiences. If the health care organization is in a particularly competitive market and loses a substantial customer, the resulting stress on the organization can be severe. This stress, like that to the physiological system, can cause behavioral reactions that may be different from those expected.

Management behavior is the last, but not least, important factor that affects the dynamics of organization life. All the variables we have looked at are powerful forces operating in an organization. However, it is management behavior that can be the most powerful of all. Action will speak louder than all the espoused values and organizational mission statements. A manager's behavior acts as living proof of what the organization wants and expects from its staff members. The issue of congruency is critical in management behavior. If a manager's behavior is congruent with the stage of growth, values, mission/goals, and systems of the organization, it is almost certain that the behavioral outcomes will match expectations. If there is incongruence in this chain of variables, the actions of the organization and its managers will speak louder than all the words used.

Putting This All Together through the Eyes of the Manager

This chapter has been written to explain the forces at play inside organizations and their relationships. As a manager, you can control and affect some of these forces to create a working environment that will produce the behavioral outcomes you desire. You can create mini organizations with their own stages of growth and behavioral characteristics. You can also express values and mission statements that your own department or section can represent. You may not always have a hand in the development of psychological and technical systems, but you may have an impact on how those systems are used. The external competition and its impact may or may not be out of your control, but you can have a better understanding of how that variable creates stress in the organization and can consequently manage some of its repercussions. Ultimately, this chapter is reduced to two simple organizational theories. One, there are a number of variables that affect organization life and staff member behaviors. The more congruent they are with each other, the easier it will be to understand and manage. Two, as a manager you are one of the most powerful variables in this dynamic chain. How you behave can and does make a difference.

Robert Inguagiato, MBA, is Executive Vice President, Temenos, Inc., a management consulting firm in Honolulu, Hawaii.

CHAPTER 3

The Roles and Responsibilities of Clinical Department Heads

by Charles E. Hollerman, MD, FACPE

Introduction

The roles of clinical department heads will vary according to a number of factors, including but not limited to:

The size of the hospital[1]
In a recent survey of hospitals ranging in size from 50 to more than 600 beds, the responsibilities of the clinical department head included quality assurance and supervision of physicians in all. However, responsibilities for budget development, recruitment, and supervision of other employees were added as the size of the hospital increased.

Whether the hospital is a teaching or a nonteaching institution.
If the hospital is a teaching institution (defined as being involved in medical student or residency training programs), the clinical department head's role will depend on whether it is a community teaching, nonuniversity-affiliated hospital; a community teaching, university-affiliated institution, or a university-based teaching hospital. The institutional designation may also result in different priorities in relation to patient care, education, research, and administration. In all hospitals, high-quality patient care is obviously a prime attribute. However, in teaching hospitals, and especially in university institutions, the attainment of high-quality patient care is derived from an emphasis on education and research that then enhances patient care. In a nonteaching hospital, patient care might be the sole attribute, whereas in a community teaching hospital, patient care is primary, with teaching relegated to a secondary role and research a distant third. In all institutions, the administrative role is integral to accomplishing the departmental goals and objectives.

15

The method of selection of the department head.
In perhaps the majority of hospitals, department heads are elected by members of the department. The term of office may be two years, and they may be able to succeed themselves. In other hospitals they may be full-time employees of the hospital, appointed by administration, with the approval of the governing board. The length of tenure in office in such instances may be defined by contract, and the roles of department head may be beyond those usually found in medical staff by-laws.

The medical staff structure.
The traditional medical staff model is structured along divisional (departmental) lines, e.g., medicine, surgery, pediatrics, etc., with subspecialty sections within each major department (or in some instances with a subspecialty, e.g., neurology, being a separate department). Other models, however, do exist. One author[2] has delineated three alternative models:

✦ The independent-corporate model, in which the medical staff is totally independent.

✦ The divisional model, of which there are three variants. One variant is based on the integration of major functional areas within medical divisions (departments), an arrangement sometimes referred to as the "Hopkins Model."[3,4] In this model, hospital functional areas, such as nursing, finance, planning, marketing, housekeeping, etc., are included within each department and report to the head of the department. Alternatively, there could be divisional models structured into such areas as primary care, maternal-child health, chronic diseases, and so on, or along product/services lines, such as oncology, cardiovascular, neurological, etc. In all the divisional models, the functional hospital areas are integral to the division. In the nontraditional divisional models, the role of the department head becomes blurred or nonexistent. Many of the traditional roles of the department head, such as quality assessment and credentialing, are performed by the division itself.

✦ In the third alternative model, a medical staff organization is developed that runs parallel to the traditional medical staff structure. This structure is directed by a steering committee composed of both hospital and medical staff members. Examples given of such parallel organization include IPAs, joint ventures, and physician-hospital associations.

In some hospitals today, there are examples of all of the above alternative models developing and/or coexisting with the traditional medical staff organization.

The positional relationship(s) with the president/chief of medical staff, a medical director, and/or the dean of a medical school.
There is virtually always an elected leader of the medical staff. In increasing numbers, there are also medical directors whose function may be purely liaison between the medical staff, administration, and the board, or may include operational duties. The latter usually includes direction of quality management and

utilization review staff, as well as administrative direction of the medical staff office. However, there are operational areas being added, including direct reporting and budgetary authority for clinical departments, as well as medical support areas such as admissions and medical records. In university hospitals, the head of the department is usually the head of the associated medical school department and directly reports to the dean of the school of medicine. Within that framework, the head of the department may also be responsible for directing an associated faculty practice plan. Such plans are also being developed in teaching, nonuniversity affiliated hospitals. In teaching hospitals with full-time faculty, the head of the department takes on an additional duty: managing "town-gown" interactions. A recent article describes the transition from a voluntary hospital to a teaching hospital with full-time compensated faculty.[5] The specter of the leadership and control of the medical staff being assumed by paid department heads, resulting in an evolution to a predicted full-time multispecialty group practice is highlighted in the article.

Despite the organizational diversity and complexity described above, one author has described a key functional role for the department head[6]: "be a 'communications expert'—amplify and translate the needs of the department into language that is understandable by those governing the institution; at the same time chairmen must interpret and communicate institutional and strategic goals to their departmental colleagues." The reader is referred to other articles expanding upon the diversity of roles in a variety of institutional settings.[6-13] This chapter will attempt to review, within broad categories, the common roles of department heads, primarily within the traditional medical staff model. These categories will not follow the outline of responsibilities typically contained in medical staff by-laws.[14] The chapter will conclude with an overview of the relationships that may exist between the department head and other managers, especially the medical director.

Roles (Duties and Responsibilities)

Quality Improvement and Credentialing

These intertwined responsibilities constitute a significant role for the department head in virtually all institutions. The term quality improvement is used rather than the prior terms of quality assurance or quality assessment. Some would use the term "total quality management" (TQM), of which continuous quality improvement (CQI) is a component; others would have CQI be premiere. It is not the purpose of this chapter to review the changes occurring in the area of quality management; the reader is referred to selected publications[15-20] on that topic; it is also discussed in this monograph in Chapter 12.

The following captures the essence of the department head's role in these areas:

✦ Be accountable for all professional, educational, and administrative activities within the department, particularly those related to the quality of patient care rendered by members of the department, and for the effective implementation of the hospital's continuous quality improvement program and other quality improvement functions delegated to the department.

✦ Develop and implement short- and long-term departmental plans that include incorporation in the credentialing and privileging process for members of the department an evaluation of individual quality improvement activities, utilization of resources, and continuing medical education, as well as evidence of appropriate professional conduct and competency. Specifically, this means the department head has responsibility for appointment, reappointment, and granting of clinical privileges, including evaluation of the applicant/department member's professional competence, conduct, and cost-effective practice of medicine. In the appointment process, the department head must focus on:

— The preapplication process (where one exists).

— The application process, particularly in regard to verifying information, gathering references, and interviewing applicants. In most hospitals, verifying information and obtaining references is the responsibility of the medical staff office, often under the direction of a medical director. However, the department head must analyze the data and the applicant and provide a recommendation. This role cannot and should not be delegated to a committee or to the department as a whole. Such delegation may raise questions related to antitrust or economic competition.

— Delineation of privileges. The department head must be satisfied that the applicant has the prerequisite training and experience to perform the privileges requested. Assistance from subspecialty division chiefs is appropriate when the clinical area is outside the department head's expertise; nevertheless, the department head is accountable for validating the applicant's competence.

The department head is also responsible for developing criteria for clinical privileges. Today, interdepartmental negotiation to establish criteria for privileges that cross traditional departmental lines is common. Aid in establishing such criteria is available.[21]

— Monitoring the applicant's performance. The initial appointment is often termed provisional or probationary for a period. While the applicant is in that status, the department head should arrange for monitoring of the appointee's performance in terms of competence as well as professional conduct.

In the reappointment process, examination of the quality aspects of the practitioner's care is mandated. The Joint Commission on Accreditation of Healthcare Organizations (JCAHO) requires documentation that reappointment decisions are based on measurement of quality and on a review of the care provided by the appointee since the prior appointment/reappointment period.[22] The hospital, through its quality management staff and/or medical staff office, should provide staff support for this role of the department head; however, the data requirements and the analysis are the responsibility of the department head.

The ultimate responsibility for quality of care, for appointments to the medical staff, and for credentialing for clinical privileges resides with the governing board. However, the board delegates the process to the medical staff, which in turn holds the department head accountable.

A major controversy is developing nationwide in one area of credentialing—namely "economic credentialing."[23,24] As noted previously, one role of the department head is to evaluate the appointee's cost-efficient practice of medicine. This provision raises the specter of "economic credentialing." What is intended is that the practitioner deliver high-quality patient care without under- or overutilization of resources. Disquality of care includes such factors as unnecessary surgery, unnecessary laboratory tests or x-rays, incorrect treatment, or improper prescriptions. These and other aspects of quality-cost relationships are discussed in an article outlining a generic model of these relationships in health care.[25] The point is that one should not be credentialed on the basis of economic factors in absentia. Quality of care must be paramount, but efficient use of resources should be considered. There are only finite resources that must be shared among many patients.

General Medical Staff Affairs
The following delineate the role of the department head in general medical staff affairs:

✦ Conduct monthly departmental meetings to discuss programs and changes in policy and to conduct review of professional services and educational activities. The departmental meetings may be conducted in two parts: business and quality management. The latter is a review required by the JCAHO. It directly relates to the areas of quality improvement and credentialing discussed above. The business meeting involves the "communications expert" role described in the Introduction. Further, it is at this meeting that long-range plans for proper growth, expansion, and diversification of the department can be discussed and prepared for implementation. A major role for the department head in these meetings is to manage change: change in departmental direction, change in quality measurement, change in hospital-medical staff relations.

✦ Enforce the hospital and medical staff by-laws, rules, regulations and policies within the department, including initiating corrective action and investigation of the practitioner's clinical performance and determining whether consultations were ordered when necessary. The major roles played in this arena are those of enforcer, disciplinarian, and investigator. This area includes identifying impaired physicians, counseling disruptive physicians, and dealing with complaints, such as sexual harassment. Policies for dealing with all these issues should be contained in the medical staff by-laws. However, the department head bears the major responsibility for investigating incidents and carrying out corrective action.

✦ Be a member of the medical executive committee, give guidance for the overall medical policies of the hospital, and make specific recommendations and suggestions regarding his or her own department and divisions. This role has been deemed legislative by some.[10] The department head has the responsibility to provide input into the overall medical policy/operation of the hospital. This role is usually delineated in medical staff by-laws. It includes quality measurement, credentialing, and corrective actions previously outlined.

✦ Establish and periodically review and revise plans for the effective emergency operation of the department in the event of an institutional or community-wide disaster. The accomplishment of this role requires interdepartmental and intrainstitutional collaboration. No single department is capable of providing all the activities in a disaster. This role mandates that the department head be a team player, not an autonomous entity.

General/Administrative/Hospital Affairs
Staff development may consist of two components:

✦ Medical staff development in the organizational sense of recruitment and retention of appropriate physicians to further the breadth and depth of patient care.

✦ Development of individual medical staff members, e.g., for leadership roles.

Recruitment should be consistent with the hospital's and the department's goals and in accordance with the medical staff by-laws and medical staff development plan. This role may be shared with the medical director or with another administration/board designee responsible for the medical staff development plan. The department head should be aware of the physicians who are being recruited by members of his or her department. Additionally, through departmental meetings, the department head should be working with department members to identify new programs/services that, in concert with the hospital's plan, would entail the recruitment of physicians with disciplines and/or skills similar to or different from those of physicians currently on the medical staff. The department chair has the responsibility to communicate departmental recommendations and to express its views to administration.

The department head also has an obligation to the department, the hospital, and individual medical staff members to assist in the development of departmental members' abilities. This role may simply call for identifying potential leaders. It may involve being a mentor, or it may involve counseling an appointee on available avenues for personal/professional growth.

If the department head has budget responsibility, the administrative role that is required in such circumstances includes:

✦ Preparation and implementation of business and marketing plans based on approved strategic plans.

✦ Formulation, justification, and administration of the departmental budget in accordance with institutional policies and departmental goals.

✦ Management of human and fiscal resources of the department to maximize achievements in service, as well as in teaching and research if within a teaching hospital.

✦ Cooperation and collaboration with other hospital departments and with hospital administration in matters affecting patient care, including personnel, supplies, standing orders, and techniques.

Paperwork is an accompaniment of the role of the department head. Generally, reports need to be provided to designated hospital administrative staff, usually the medical director if there is one, regarding departmental activities and strategy. Annual departmental reports also are routinely required by the president of the medical staff and, although not usually in the same format, by the medical director, hospital president, or the board. Being a "communication expert" requires skills in both verbal and written presentation.

Education and Research
If the institution is involved in teaching and/or research, the department head role includes the following duties and responsibilities:

✦ Serve as, or select, program director of associated residency program.

✦ Lead and guide members of the department in developing, maintaining, and enhancing intra- and interdepartmental educational programs that support high academic standards, are current, and are responsive to learners' needs.

✦ Lead and guide members of the department in establishing high, but realistic, goals for intra- and interdepartmental research programs in relation to such factors as staff expertise, availability of funding, needs for equipment, availability of space, and number of support personnel needed.

✦ Submit and have articles accepted in peer-reviewed publications.

✦ Aid in identifying funding sources—both public and private—for both instruction and research; encourage grant applications and the cultivation of private donors.

✦ Be responsible for ensuring that departmental member are aware of and in compliance with institutional policies and procedures in the conduct of research.

Institutional and Community Relations
The department head is expected to be a role model within the department, the medical staff, the hospital, and the community. This role carries with it the obligation to carry out the duties and responsibilities of the position in a manner consistent with the vision, mission, goals, and values of the institution. Further, there is a responsibility to the community to promote service by members of the department. Additionally, as a role model, the department head must show leadership in his or her chosen field; this could include service on relevant task forces or committees at the institutional, local, state, regional, or national levels.

The majority of department heads, elected or appointed, do carry out many of these responsibilities of a role model.

Relation to Other Hospital Managers

The relation of the department head to other hospital managers, including the medical director, will depend on the organizational structure of the hospital. In some institutions, the department head will be the leader of the management team, for example in the divisional models mentioned in the introduction. The much more likely relationship, however, will be that of being a team member. The latter position is not a familiar or comfortable one for many physicians, because they are accustomed to being the "captain of the ship." No one person, no one department, can provide the answers to the cross-disciplinary issues that exist in today's health care institutions—indeed, it is unlikely that such was ever the case. The department head must thus work in a collaborative fashion with other hospital managers to accomplish the goals of the hospital as well as those of the department. Suppose, for example, the head of an emergency department wishes to have patients admitted in a more timely manner. That admission process will depend, at least, upon registrars, medical records personnel, ancillary departments such as radiology and laboratory medicine providing expeditious turnaround times on x-rays and tests, escort personnel, housekeeping providing "ready" beds, and floor nurses able and willing to accept patients. The accomplishment of the department head's desire demands the input and involvement of a variety of services. The department head cannot just order it to be accomplished.

In general terms, the department head's relationship with the medical director encompasses information sharing, i.e., two-way communication. The department head should keep the medical director apprised of department/medical staff needs and concerns, as well as recommend proposals for changes. Conversely, the medical director should not only keep the department head aware of the plans and decisions of administration that will affect the department, but also serve as a link between department heads. Further, the medical director is most likely the hospital person held accountable for overall medical quality improvement and credentialing. In the area of quality, the medical director provides oversight and direction. In the area of credentialing, the medical director must often serve as staff to the department head. The medical director, through the medical staff office, assembles all the information required for appointment/reappointment, which is then provided to the department head for analysis and recommendation. In situations where the department head manages the budget and reports to a medical director, the latter is responsible for overseeing budget formulation, implementation, and monitoring.

Finally, the department head's relationship to the president/chief of the medical staff is usually through the medical executive committee and other committees of the medical staff. The president/chief of staff is responsible for ensuring that the by-laws of the medical staff are adhered to. The department heads are, therefore, accountable to the president/chief of staff in carrying out the by-laws requirements.

Projections

It is likely that the future will see more full-time medical directors and department heads. At a minimum, there will be an increase in part-time positions, with compensation for administrative duties. The clinical linkage with the administrative activities of the hospital will be the major factor in the success of hospitals. The department head can no longer be selected on the basis of being a nice person, willing to do the job, or a superb clinician. The selection, whether by election or appointment, must be based on administrative skills that are in balance with clinical and political skills. Obviously, in teaching institutions educational and/or research skills would be added qualifications.

Summary

In reviewing the material presented in this chapter, one can see that the roles of the department head include being, first and foremost, a leader and communicator. However, other roles depend on the situation and circumstances, e.g., arbitrator, negotiator, enforcer, counselor, disciplinarian, innovator, advocate (for both patient and organization), visionary, change agent, influencer, planner, evaluator, ad infinitum. In a word, the department head is a *manager*; in two words, a *physician manager* who is an interface professional,[26,27] whether employed or voluntary. This requires the attainment of new skills—management skills—so the department head can provide effective leadership within the hospital community.

References

1. Curry, W. "Hospital Size Determines Department Director Policy." *Physician Executive* 16(6):24-5, Nov.-Dec. 1990.

2. Shortell, S. "The Medical Staff of the Future: Replanting the Garden." *Frontiers of Health Services Management* 1(3):3-48, Feb. 1985.

3. Heyssel, R., and others. "Decentralized Management in a Teaching Hospital." *New England Journal of Medicine* 310(22):1477-80, May 31, 1984.

4. Brady, T., and Carpenter, C. "Defining the Management Role of the Departmental Medical Director." *Hospital and Health Services Administration* 31(5):69-85, Sept.-Oct. 1986.

5. Davis, W. "One Community Hospital—2000 A.D." *Physician Executive* 16(2):31-2, Mar.-Apr. 1990.

6. Popp, A. "The Neurosurgeon as a Chairman of Surgery." *Surgery Neurology* 31(2):92-5, Feb. 1989.

7. McKhann, G. "Clinical Department Manager: Manager or Scholar." *Annals of Neurology* 26(61):779-81, Dec. 1989.

8. Betson, C., and Pedroja, A. "Physician Managers: A Description of Their Job in Hospitals." *Hospital and Health Services Administration* 34(3):353-69, Fall 1989.

9. Johnson, E. "Managing Physician-Directed Departments. *Hospital and Health Services Administration* 24(3):96-101, Summer 1979.

10. Angermeier, I., and Booth, R. "Establishing an Appropriate Role for Physician Involvement in Hospital Department Operations." *Hospital and Health Services Administration* 28(6):59-76, Nov.-Dec. 1983.

11. Dallman, J. "Hospital Department Chief—Administrator or Brother's Keeper?" *Hospital Physician* 24(15):13,17, May 1988.

12. Walt, A. "The Surgical Chairmanship in a Corporate World." *Archives of Surgery* 123(7):805-9, July 1988.

13. Mayer, T. "The Emergency Department Medical Director." *Emergency Clinics of North America* 5(1):1-29, Feb. 1987.

14. *By-Laws—A Guide for Hospital Medical Staffs.* Chicago, Ill.: American Medical Association, 1984, pp. 37-38.

15. Berwick, D. "Continuous Improvement as an Ideal in Health Care." *New England Journal of Medicine* 320(1):53-6, Jan. 5, 1989.

16. McLaughlan, C., and Kaluzny, A. "Total Quality Management in Health: Making It Work." *Health Care Management Review* 15(3):7-14, Summer, 1990.

17. Merry, M. "Total Quality Management for Physicians: Translating the new Paradigm." *QRB* 16(3):101-5, March 1990.

18. O'Leary, D. "Accreditation in the Quality Improvement Mold—A Vision for Tomorrow." *QRB* 17(3):72-7, March 1991.

19. Laffel, G., and Blumenthal, D. "The Case for Using Industrial Quality Management Science in Health Care Organizations." *JAMA* 262(20):2869-73, Nov. 24, 1989.

20. Marszalek-Gaucher, E., and Coffey, R. *Transforming Healthcare Organizations: How to Achieve and Sustain Organizational Excellence.* San Francisco, Calif.: Jossey-Bass, Publishers, 1990.

21. "Current Challenges in Delineating Clinical Privileges." *The Quality Letter for Healthcare Leaders* 2(10):1-16, Dec. 1990-Jan. 1991.

22. *Accreditation Manual for Hospitals.* Oakbrook Terrace, Ill.: Joint Commission on Accreditation of Healthcare Organizations, 1991, pp. 216-7.

23. Lang, H. "Economic Credentialing—Why It Must Be Stopped." *The Medical Staff Counselor* 5(2):19-25, Spring 1991.

24. Greene, J. "System Pioneers Credentialing." *Modern Heathcare* 21(17):32-4,36, April 29, 1991.

25. Klint, R., and Long, H. "Cost/Quality Relationship: A Generic Model for Health Care." In *New Leadership in Health Care Management: The Physician Executive,* Curry, W., Editor, Tampa, Fla: American College of Physician Executives, 1988, pp. 159-75.

26. Kaiser, L. "Key Management Skills for the Physician Executive." In *New Leadership in Health Care Management: The Physician Executive*, Curry, W., Editor. Tampa, Fla.: American College of Physician Executives, 1988, pp. 78-101.

27. Cordes, D., and others. "Management Roles for Physicians: Training Residents for the Reality." *Journal of Occupational Medicine* 30(1):863-7, Nov. 1988.

Charles E. Hollerman, MD, FACPE, is Vice President, Medical Affairs, St. Joseph's Mercy Hospitals and Health Services, Mt. Clemens, Michigan.

CHAPTER 4

Effective Communication

by Barbara J. Linney, MA

*T*he role of the chief of service and department chair varies from organization to organization, but it is always a physician who has been thrust into a leadership role. Whatever the specifics of their roles, chief of service and department chairs have to be able to communicate effectively with a vide array of individuals and groups—administrators, doctors, other department leaders, nurses, and the public, to name a few.

The chief of neurology may want to convince the administration that his or her department is the best one to run the sleep lab. The chairman of obstetrics and gynecology may need to convince physicians in the department to cooperate and adhere to surgical standards. If someone is doing hysterectomies that do not meet prescribed criteria, the department and the hospital will be in trouble with regulators. The chief of orthopedics may need to talk to the head of physical therapy about procedures in that department. The chief is not that person's boss, an assistant administrator is, so he or she would need to tactfully make suggestions, not give orders, to get things done. The chair of obstetrics needs to cooperate with the chair of pediatrics because the departments often share the same patients.

Robert Thornton, MD, a neurologist in Winter Park, Florida, has said that chiefs or chairs are the first ones to get requests from outside sources to make talks to the public, often on television, or to write concise, understandable articles on conditions such as stroke, epilepsy, and heart disease. "If you don't do it, your competition will. It is the best and least expensive source of referrals."[1]

Good communication is needed in all these situations. The main skills needed for good communication are talking so that people will want to listen to you, listening so that people will want to talk to you, and writing so that people will want to read what you have written.

There are ways to improve these skills and enable communication to take place. If someone absolutely does not want to communicate with you, nothing will work. It takes two people putting forth energy for a good interaction to happen, but if you will work on your techniques, you will find more people will respond to you in a positive way.

Talking

What will make people listen to you when you talk?

+ **Pronounce your words clearly.** Enunciate. Don't mumble. You need to use the energy to project your voice to the other person. He or she should not have to strain to hear you. It is very annoying to try to have a conversation with someone you cannot hear or understand. But neither should you yell at them.

+ **Don't talk too quickly or too slowly.** Southerners sometimes have to speed up. Northerners sometimes have to slow down. Midwesterners usually have it about right.

+ **Look at the other person.** Look as if you are enjoying the conversation. You don't have to stare the person down, but if your eyes wander all over the room or you always look over their shoulders, listeners have a hard time paying attention to what you are saying. They secretly speculate about what you are looking at rather than listening to what you are saying.

+ **Use average size words.** If you sling a lot of jargon or large words that most people do not know, you alienate them. Patients do not know what MRI or myocardial infarction means.

+ **Don't talk longer than a couple of minutes without letting the other person talk.** Taking turns was a valuable thing to learn in preschool, and we never outgrow the need to do it. As a shy child, I didn't always get my turn, and I felt sad, left out, angry. Sometimes I'd go away feeling lonely. Other times I'd try to figure out how to get revenge, particularly with my older brother. Using Jung's concept of extrovert and introvert, extroverts talk and then figure out what they think; introverts figure out what they think and then talk. The introverts have valuable information if you give them time to say it. It's the job of any physician executive to be sure he or she gets ideas from both kinds, or unneeded resentment builds in the organization. It requires restraining the quick talkers some and encouraging those who do not speak up quickly.

+ **Be willing to tell what you feel about a subject as well as what you think.** Give a personal example. "I think we would have better meetings with the doctors if we met at 6 p.m. instead of 9 p.m. Frankly, I'm just too tired to concentrate at 9 p.m. after I've worked a 12-hour shift."

✦ **Avoid teasing.** People fear others will humiliate them for the way they look, for what they say, or for what they have done. They cope with this fear in several ways. Some try to talk a lot and thus control the words. If they are doing the talking, they may not be hurt by someone else's words. Others do not speak up for fear of saying something wrong and not being able to come back with a defense.

Teasing can be fun between equals, but often it is a secret form of aggression, and it strips its victim of power unless both parties are equally good at the quick barb. Teasing usually allows the one doing the teasing to feel one up. This occasionally feels good, but it eliminates closeness and builds resentment. A doctor's teasing nurses is not good unless nurses feel equally free to tease the doctor. The latter is rare. If you tease your children a lot, you may want to rethink that. You are not equals. The child usually feels very bad, even though he or she may be laughing.

✦ Don't overuse big emotions, such as anger or tears. There are times when we are angry and the other person must know it, but those times are rare. It's similar to the little boy who hollered "wolf." If you are crying or angry in most of your exchanges, no one will listen or take you seriously. People will learn to tune you out or will automatically scream back at you.

Big emotions usually interfere with communication. The listener is often threatened, frightened, or repulsed by a show of uncontrolled emotion, and he or she cannot hear the words being spoken. The person raging or crying also cannot hear when the listener responds.

What can you do when emotions are raging?

When you are the speaker, "Writing in [a] journal about people or situations that have evoked in us anger, anxiety, or a sense of defeat helps to stabilize our psychological situation and strengthen our ego. It helps us to 'get a handle' on our emotions without repressing them, and to get a look at the giant that threatens to swallow us. If we do this before we get into a discussion that might become highly emotional, the chances are good that we can express our feelings to the other person and not be consumed by them."[2]

When you are the listener, if you are feeling strong and collected, it is helpful if you can let the emotional person vent for a few moments. You might then respond, "I can see that you are angry, and I'm not surprised. What can I do to help?" If you are not up to being in the presence of so much negative energy, you might say, "I'll be glad to talk about this when you are calmer."

✦ Know what you want. It is a good idea to prepare for important conversations. By writing ahead of time, you can clearly focus on what you want and on what price you are willing to pay to get it. The following questions can help you think through an important interaction ahead of time. It is not cheating to prepare; it is wise.

What do you think about the situation?
What do you feel about the situation?
What do you want?
What will be the good or bad consequences if you get it?
What are you willing to do to get what you want?
What do you think the other person wants?
Can you give any of what he or she wants?

The following is an example of using these questions. I was in the middle of a business interaction between two friends of mine. They did not know each other. Bill wanted Joe to put on a program for a group he was in. Bill was outraged at the price Joe asked and wanted me to pass a nasty message back to Joe.

What do you think about the situation? I think Bill got angry when I would not do something he asked me to do. I would not call Joe and tell him that instead of Bill's paying him to speak, Joe would have to pay Bill's group thousands of dollars for it to even let him speak to it.

What do you feel about the situation? At first I felt angry. Now I feel hurt by the rejection. Bill has not talked to me for three months.

What do you want? To have lunch together occasionally, to talk, and to share ideas but not to have him start trying to tell me outlandish things to do again.

What will be the good or bad consequences if you get what you want? Good—I'd have his stimulating mind spurring thoughts in me again. Bad—He'd get into the bossiness again, or I'd get tired of laughing at his jokes, if we had too much contact.

What are you willing to do to get what you want? Call him and say, "Could we have lunch and talk about why we don't talk anymore?" What do you think the other person wants? To be one up. Maybe an apology. I'm not sure what he wants— that's what I could find out if we talked.

Can you give him any of what he wants? I can apologize and say I didn't handle the situation well, but I can't be in a friendship where he slips into giving me orders.

✦ Use good body language. How you say something and how you look when you say it are as important as what you say. What causes someone to understand you and respond well to you? Psychologist Albert Mehrabian suggests that 7 percent of understanding depends on the words you use, 38 percent depends on your tone of voice, and 55 percent depends on your nonverbal body language.[3]

Facial expression and voice communicate much more than you realize. A listener understands and interprets your message more through the tone of your voice and the look of your body than through your words. "No, I'm not angry!" said harshly conveys the message that you are angry. "I really love that!" said sarcastically implies that you don't like it at all. People complain about getting mixed signals when the words, tone of voice, and body language send different messages. They will believe the tone of your voice and the look on your face much more than the words you say.

Alexander claims people have a hard time accepting these facts. "The reality is that few people accept responsibility for anything more than their words. They have never learned that a harsh tone can deny the gentlest of words...."[4] Most people refuse to believe it if they are the ones doing the talking, but they quickly believe it if someone else is doing the talking.

A positive voice is cheerful, satisfied, concerned, warm. A negative voice is sarcastic, scared, depressed, clipped, tense, too loud or soft. A positive face has a smile, an occasional head nod, and eye contact. A negative face has a frown, smirk, or boring glare. A positive body is relaxed, leaning forward some, with open arms. Negative body language is pointing, wandering eyes, picking at body.[5]

Listening

"...in both business and personal relationships, the consequence of inadequate listening are extraordinarily costly. Simple listening mistakes cost the business world millions of dollars annually."[6]

Most people have heard of Parent Effectiveness Training and the active listening that it recommends. Active listening has gotten some bad press, because people have overused the term, "I hear what you are saying." Also, if someone is rampaging, and I say, "You seem to be angry," a natural response might be, "You're damned right I'm angry." Active listening is a good technique, but how and when you use it needs to vary if you do not want to further alienate the person you are talking to.

"Active listening involves a restatement of either the message or the feeling of the speaker without giving advice, analyzing, or probing."[7] It is the place to begin when listening to someone with a problem. You do not want to quickly interrupt and say, "I know how you feel" or give advice. But you do not want to overdo active listening either, because the listener may feel that you are acting like a parrot or a robot.

Listening is an art that starts with attentive silence. When my children were young, if I did not look at them when they talked to me, they would say, "Turn your face, Mama." Shortly after they could talk, they knew I had to be looking at them to really be paying attention. Adults know this, too, whether they tell you or not. It's your job to hold your eyes and body so that others know you are paying attention.

Young children talk a lot, so when I couldn't listen anymore, I said so and told them I would listen more later. We need to deal with adults in the same way. If you cannot pay attention, say, "I'm swamped with this project right now, but I can give you my undivided attention at 3 p.m. Could you come back then?" Then be sure to give them the time at 3 p.m.

Try not to make a habit of pretending to listen when you are not. People will come to distrust you. However, all of us have been in long meetings when listening simply was not in us anymore. At that point, pretending to listen is better than throwing your arms back with a deep sigh or closing your eyes in a bored slouch. Such behavior has a negative effect on those who may still be paying attention.

Listening is hard work. "While an average speech rate for many people is about 200 words per minute, most of us can think about four times that speed. With all that extra think time, the ineffective listener lets his mind wander. His brain takes excursions to review the events of yesterday, or plan tomorrow, or solve a business problem...or sleep."[8] You have to work to control your mind and make it concentrate on what is being said. If you are troubled by an impending malpractice suit, a divorce, or a child who is having problems, your capacity to listen will diminish drastically. You will need to be patient with yourself in those circumstances and perhaps say to the person speaking, "I am a bit distracted. Can you tell me that again."

If you decide you are willing to expend the energy to listen, here are some techniques that will help you listen so people will want to talk to you:

+ **Be quiet.** You cannot be listening if you are talking or you are thinking hard about what you are going to say next. If you get very anxious about not knowing what to say when they finish, try putting all your energy into listening and then tell them, "I need to think about this. Can I get back with you in a while to talk more?"

+ **Use your body to let the person know you are there.** Look at him or her. Don't let your eyes wander all over the room. Sit attentively but not tensely, not slouching or lying down. On the sofa watching television or reading the paper is not a good positions for listening. Neither is opening your mail in your office while someone tries to tell you something.

+ **Give an occasional "uh huh" or nod to let people know you are following their train of thought.** If you are not, ask them a question before you let them go on too long, and you are really lost.

+ **Ask nonjudgmental questions.** "Can you say a little more? I'm not sure I understand. Will you try me again?" Don't ask, "Why on earth did you do that?" There is absolutely no decent answer to that question, and the person doing the asking is implying, "You are an idiot!" You may be right, but if you want communication to continue, you will have to discipline yourself not to say everything you think.

✦ **Restate some of what the person has said.** "Let me see if I understand. You think Dr. X is showing up for his emergency department shift with alcohol on his breath."

✦ **Make a guess about a feeling you think the person is having if it seems appropriate.** "I can see why that would make you sad." They may reply, "I'm not sad, I'm angry." It doesn't matter that you are wrong. They will correct you, and you have gotten to a deeper level of communication when you find out how someone feels about a subject. The person will feel a sense of relief and sometimes release when he or she identifies the feeling.

It is not easy to listen. We would all rather be the center of attention, doing all the talking. This is not a bad fact, just a fact. But if we do not learn to take turns, if we do not learn to listen, we will not have a chance of being heard.

Conflict

Many people would claim they do behave in ways that make interpersonal communication go more smoothly, but they also might admit that when situations get hostile, they forget everything and often react in ways that they don't like. Confrontation is difficult. People usually deal with it in one of two ways. They verbally attack, using the energy of anger to spur them on, or they withdraw, say nothing, and often plot revenge.

Confronting someone in a calm, firm voice takes courage. I'd like to suggest a how-to process that may help you control yourself if you tend to explode and may help you get the nerve to confront if you tend to withdraw. I mentioned earlier that it is helpful to prepare for important conversations. That is especially true if you are in a heated situation. Try filling in the blanks in this short formula:

When you (do so and so),
I feel (or react in this way),
Because (I think something).
I'd like you to (do so and so).

Examples:

When you verbally attack me and defend your position when I ask you to do something,
I get angry and I avoid telling you what you need to hear,
Because I think nothing will be accomplished and I dread your reaction.
Next time, I'd like you to listen until I finish and think about it, and then we can discuss it.

When you come to me with every emergency department problem you have,
I feel angry,

Because I can only deal with one dying person at a time.
I'd like you to make some of the decisions yourself. I trust your judgment.

Sometimes you take the process a step further and tell what the consequences will be if behavior is not changed.

When you leave your charts unreviewed for two weeks, the rest of the staff and I are frustrated (angry),
Because we can't properly take care of patients and get our work done.
I want you to complete them in three days. If not, I'll alert the medical records committee.

Using the formula, continue to write to find out exactly what you want to say. When you actually speak to the person, the formula will take a slightly different form. The following is what I might actually tell the person concerning the first example:

Sometimes I need to ask you to change a behavior. When I do, you quickly defend your position and verbally attack me. As a result, I dread telling you something. I put it off and yet I know you are going to suffer in your performance evaluation if you do not change. In the future, when I have something difficult to tell you, I'm going to say, "I have something difficult to tell you. " I'd like you to listen until I finish and think about it, and then we can get together to discuss it.

When you get ready to talk to the person, you may not tell them exactly what you have written, but the formula can help you get clear about what aggravates you, what part you play in creating the problem, and what it is you want to happen. If you get angry, you can cuss and vent and scream on paper and then throw it away. When you spill those feelings on people, they are usually either so angry themselves or so frightened that they cannot hear what it is you want them to do. If you are the one who often withdraws from conflict, you can sometimes get the courage to speak up, because you have written out exactly what you plan to say. You don't have to have the notes with you. Your brain has thought them and seen them on paper so it will usually remember them. You can also practice saying the words out loud so that your brain will have also heard them.

Some things you discover when you are writing, you will not want to tell. For example, that you are frightened about something. You may be too vulnerable. Someone might say, "She's not tough enough to do this job. Let's get rid of her." So you don't always *tell* what you feel, but it is very important for you to *know* what you feel. When you don't know, you can continue to act in unproductive ways (e.g., as an angry or frightened little boy or girl) and wonder why life and your job are not good. When you are aware of what you feel, you can move through it and feel something often better than the first impression. When you know, you can remind yourself that you are grown, that you have options, that this person does not have your very life in his or her hands.

If writing seems too disagreeable a task, try telling all of this to a friend before you talk to the one who has annoyed you, but don't leave it there. If the information never gets back to the person who caused you the trouble, there is no chance for the situation to improve.

When someone irritates us, we want to complain to a friend because it feels good to do so. We want to vent. I do not think this human behavior will stop, but if the listener could let the talker vent for awhile and then encourage him or her to prepare to talk to the offending person, office gossip would sometimes have a productive end rather than just fueling the "poor-me" fire.

Writing

In the land of communication, there will probably come a time when you have to write. What will make people want to read what you have written?

✦ **Make it short.** We may or may not be getting lazier, with shorter attention spans, but we are all definitely busy. Even the brightest of executives want documents to be short, because they need to get through them in a hurry.

✦ **Have enough areas on a page where there are no words.** Do you remember when, in the seventh grade, you started to read that larger geography book with more words on a page? You struggled through two columns of heavy words and then turned the page to find a picture that took up half the page. Weren't you happy, relieved? When we grow up, we pretend that we get over that thrill, but we don't. None of us want to look at a page that is heavy and mostly black with words. If there are good top, bottom, and side margins, with spaces between paragraphs and perhaps a list in the middle with more white space around it, we are invited to read what is on the page rather than repelled by it.

✦ **Avoid needless repetition.** Do not repeat the same word many times. The reader begins to hear the sing-song repetition of the word rather than your message. It is fine to repeat the same word when you are first generating your thoughts, but you need to cut them later.

Writing needs to be a two-part process. First, you come up with ideas without criticizing them at all. If you judge every word as you go, the creative part of you will get tired and will stop sending messages. Just write down or dictate the words as they come to you. Become very critical when you edit. Circle all the repeated words and try to eliminate most of them, unless you are repeating the word to emphasize its importance or changing the word would confuse the reader.

✦ **Don't be verbose.** Don't write the same idea a second time using different words: end result, final conclusion, personal opinion, unexpected surprise. Always use fewer words rather than more. "In the event that" can simply be "if." "In view of the fact that" can be "Because." Elbow says, "Every word omitted keeps another reader with you."[9] It is especially important for physicians to use simple words and phrases whenever they can because so often they must use the long technical words of their profession. Too many words of three syllables or more make for heavy reading. Resist using all you know when you want to communicate with anyone other than your medical

✦ **Use nonsexist language.** Avoid words that imply only a man or a woman could do the job. Instead of businessman, write business executive, manager, or business person. Instead of chairman say chair or chairperson. When writing to a woman, use the title "Ms." unless you know she would prefer "Mrs." or "Miss." "Mr." indicates the person you are addressing is a man but explains nothing about his marital status. "Ms." does the same for a woman. Instead of using the masculine pronoun (he, his, him) when referring to a group that includes both men and women, make the subject of the sentence plural and thus neutral. Sometimes you will have to use the singular pronoun. When you do, write "he or she" or "he/she." Too many of these sound awkward, but it is no longer acceptable to use just "he."

✦ **Always choose precise words over vague words.** Instead of "nice house" say "brick house." Instead of "circumstance" put "Hurricane Hugo." Use strong verbs rather than ones hidden in many words. "Decide" is stronger than "make a decision." "Buy" is better than "make a purchase." "Help" is clearer than "give assistance."

✦ **Don't use jargon unless you are absolutely sure the listener understands it.** Jargon, in its broadest definition, is any language that is hard to understand. Sometimes it acts as a shield for those who don't have much to say. It can be specialized vocabulary that a particular group of people understand. Teenagers find a different set of words every two or three years that, they hope, will confuse their parents. Accountants, chemists, bankers, doctors, and others have special terms that must be defined when they are working with the general public. Abbreviations that the listener does not understand are jargon. It's the writer's job to find out what the reader knows and doesn't know. When it comes to abbreviations, if you are in doubt, write it out.

Often jargon is phony, inflated, and uselessly complex. A client told me once, "If I speak and write so others understand me, they will steal my job." The opposite is more often true—jargon interferes with communication and could cause you to lose your job. People get angry if you use difficult words without explaining their meaning. They put your memos in the trash and do not do what you have asked them to do.

✦ **Avoid trite phrases.** Overworked expressions make a reader switch from paying attention to your message to being irritated that you are saying the same old thing. "The bottom line," "the whole nine yards," and "I need your input" are phrases that need a few year's rest. If you can finish the following statements, they have probably been overused.

Enclosed_____

We're sorry for any _____

It has come to our_____

Please call at your earliest_____

If you have additional questions, feel _____

Try substituting new words. Examples for the first and second phrases might be, "Here is the information you asked for in your letter of June 5," and "Thanks for your patience with this delay."[10]

✦ **Tone or manner of expression is as evident in the written word as it is in the spoken word.** Business correspondence used to have a stuffy, legalistic tone. Now companies like a conversational, friendly tone that sounds as if a person, not a machine, wrote the letter. Pretend the reader is standing beside you. If you wouldn't say "per your request" to his or her face, don't write it in the letter.

Use a positive tone whenever possible. "Saying that someone is 'interested in details' conveys a more positive tone than saying the individual is a 'nitpicker.' The word economical is more positive than stingy or cheap."[11]

I've given you several do's and don't's, but what if you hate the whole writing process. Is there anything that would make you dread it less? The answer is writing more, but in a different way. Write 10 minutes a day, five days a week, on any subject that pops into your head. Use a kind of paper and pen that you like or type it on a word processor if that's easier for you. (Whatever paper or instrument you decide to write on I'll now refer to as your journal). Don't worry about spelling, punctuation, grammar, or anything that some English teacher told you to worry about. There is just one catch—you must start writing and not stop until the time is up. If you can't think of anything to write, just write, "I can't think of anything. I can't think of anything. This is one of the dumbest things I've ever done," but keep writing. Ideas will pop into your head if you keep writing that simply will not occur to you if you just sit and think.

If you were going to run in a 10 kilometer race on the weekend, you would need to do some daily running to get ready. The same is true for writing. You need to grease the machinery of your hand and brain to make them readily give you words when you need to write something.

This writing exercise will not only make the writing process easier but also can enhance your verbal communication skills and benefit you in other ways. It can help you organize your day. You probably already make a "to do" list. Expand it. Gripe—"month end report for Mr. Jones. I hate the way he makes red marks and gives it back to me to do again just to show he has the power to do that. Performance appraisal for Dr. Thomas. QA meeting—they go on and on without making a decision." You will think of the items to do much quicker if you write comments about them as you go. When you finish the journal entry, circle the tasks that came up that need to be done that day and assign them numbers in order of importance.

Writing in a journal can help you get rid of frustration. Anger is a physical phenomenon. You feel it somewhere in your body—knotted stomach, clinched fist, stiff neck. You cannot always avoid getting angry, but you need to get it out of your system for good health, and you don't want to dump it on the wrong person. You can dump it in your journal. Peter Elbow says, "Garbage in your head will poison you. Garbage on paper can safely be put in the waste paper basket."[12]

Writing quickly without stopping taps your right brain creativity. Most of us judge our ideas quickly. As soon as they pop into our heads, we think, "That will never work. Someone will think that is stupid." If you continue to write, the censor who seems to sit on your shoulder is thwarted and cannot continue to judge every thought. Thus the right brain will keep sending you fresh thoughts because you are receiving them and showing respect by writing them down. Some of the ideas will be useful, but not all. You have to get a fair number of ideas out to have a few that are good.

While writing, you can find creative solutions to relationship problems. If you and your boss or spouse or child disagree over the same topic repeatedly, write out the scene in your journal. Often you wish you had said something differently or had not cried or had not lost your temper. Write the scene the way you wish it had happened. Next time you'll be amazed at how the interaction is similar to what you wrote, because you stayed calm in your half of the conversation.

If you decide to write in a journal, keep it hidden or tear up any incriminating evidence. Writing will take you places you didn't know you were going to go. If you momentarily hate your boss, it is helpful to write about it but harmful if anyone sees it. You do not have to keep what you write in order to benefit from having written it.

If you've recognized a communication skill you would like to improve, what activities will help you change?

✦ Practice on a friend.

✦ Practice in front of a video camera.

✦ Write about it in your journal.

✦ Put little reminder notes to yourself where no one else can see them—in your desk drawer or the medicine cabinet. Examples: I will let others have a chance to talk. I am a good listener. I am a strong energetic speaker.

✦ Relax and talk to yourself. The brain is much like a computer. It can be programmed and reprogrammed. If you don't like what you are doing, start to talk to yourself about a positive change. Learn some kind of relaxation technique. The best ones ask you to tense and release each set of muscles while breathing deeply. Do the exercise every day for three weeks. Each time you finish doing the exercise, say a positive statement to yourself about some desired change. Examples: I can control my temper. I can speak up when I choose to. The subconscious is more receptive when your body is relaxed. After several weeks, you'll be aware that you are interacting with people differently. Changing the way you communicate is not easy. It requires practicing new behavior that will feel awkward for a while, but the effort's worth it. "Nothing is more essential to success in any area of your life than the ability to communicate well. Nothing can compare to the joy of communicating love, of being heard and understood completely, of discovering some profound insight from another's mind, or of transmitting your own thoughts to a rapt audience."[13]

References

1. Thornton, R. Personal communication.

2. Sanford, J. *Between People, Communicating One-to-One.* New York, N.Y.: Paulist Press, 1982, p. 37.

3. Malandro, L., and Barker, L. *Nonverbal Communication.* Reading, Mass.: Addison-Wesley Publishing Co., 1983, p. 278.

4. Alexander, J. *Dare to Change.* New York, N.Y.: New American Library, 1984, p. 138.

5. Swets, P. *The Art of Talking So That People Will Listen.* Englewood Cliffs, N.J.: Prentice-Hall, Inc., 1983, p. 59.

6. *Ibid.,* p. 40.

7. Carr, J. *Communicating and Relating.* Menlo Park, Calif.: Benjamin/Cummings Publishing Co., Inc., 1979, p. 152.

8. Swets, P., *op. cit.,* p. 42.

9. Elbow, P. *Writing Without Teachers.* London: Oxford University Press, 1973, p. 41.

10. Laura Brill and Associates. *How to Sharpen Your Business Writing Skills.* New York, N.Y.: American Management Association, 1985.

11. Kolin, P. *Successful Writing at Work.* Lexington, Mass.: D.C. Heath and Co., 1980, p.13.

12. Elbow, P., *op. cit.,* p. 8.

13. Swets, P., *op. cit.,* p. 4.

Works consulted but not cited

Goldberg, N. *Writing Down the Bones*. Boston, Mass.: Shambala, 1986.

Gordon, T. *P.E.T.* New York, N.Y.: Peter H. Wyden, Inc., 1973.

Horton, S. *Thinking Through Writing*. Baltimore, Md.: Johns Hopkins University Press, 1982.

Klauser, H. *Writing on Both Sides of the Brain: Breakthrough Techniques for People Who Write*. San Francisco, Calif.: Harper and Row, Publishers, 1986.

Maltz, M. *Psycho-Cybernetics*. Hollywood, Calif.: Wilshire Book Co., 1960.

Milo, F. *How to Get Your Point Across in 30 Seconds-or Less*. New York, N.Y.: Simon and Schuster, 1986.

James, M., and Jongeward, D. *Born to Win*. Philippines: Addison-Wesley Publishing Co., Inc., 1971.

Barbara J. Linney, MA, is Director of Career Development for the American College of Physician Executives, Tampa, Florida.

CHAPTER 5

Negotiating Skills

by Howard E. Rotner, MD, FACPE

Introduction

Negotiation skills rank among the highest priorities for the successful physician leader. It is safe to predict that not a day will go by when, as a physician leader, you won't encounter some negotiation, large or small. Regrettably, however, many new physician leaders are extremely wary of negotiations, perceiving that participation results in exposure to unnecessary and unwanted risk. You may perceive that *relationships* that you have worked hard to build and value highly might be threatened by the fear of rancor associated with negotiation.

Moreover, lacking significant experience in formal negotiations, you may imagine that you have no business "playing with the big boys." Perhaps, you think, physician negotiations should be conducted by other members of the management team, such as the CEO, the vice president for operations, or the vice president for medical affairs. The purpose of this chapter is to dispel these ideas and allow you to become comfortable in a skill that you cannot and should not avoid. It is a skill that has the potential to considerably elevate your stature and add immeasurably to your power. The alternative is to not engage in negotiations and proportionately diminish your power. If the you see negotiations as opportunities to attain commitments never before imagined or proposed, you will enhance the fortunes of your organization many times over.

The opportunities for negotiation for the physician leader are legion. Requests for office space cannot all be accommodated. The part A contract for pathologists is being negotiated, and you know that they are being grossly overpaid according to the standards of surrounding hospitals in the area. The paid director's position of the ambulatory surgicenter has just become available, and four surgeons approach you for the position. You are attempting to recruit a large internal medicine group to use your hospital's facilities, but they are resistant thus far. Your medical records delinquencies do not fulfill JCAHO standards and your survey is coming up this year. Much of the physician leader's work is consumed by persuading other people to act in a way that meets the needs of the institution. Each of these efforts becomes, in one way or another, a negotiation. Your success is very much connected to how effective you are in the art of persuading and using negotiation skills.

Can someone else do it better?

All of us have been exposed to the necessity of negotiating on many levels throughout our lives. If you have been selected to be a physician leader in your organization, it is safe to assume that you have already achieved a record of success. Intuitively, you have negotiated on many levels, such as the purchase of your house, the salary and benefits of your job, numerous expectations and needs within your family, and agreements with your colleagues, to name just a few. On balance, it is safe to say that you have applied your knowledge, values, and convictions to arrive at fundamentally sound solutions. In your organization, there probably is no person who is more qualified to comprehend the interests of both parties, or is more interested in a principled agreement, than you. The real question is not, "Can someone else do it better?" It is, "Who can possibly negotiate better than you?"

Am I placing myself at undue risk by participating in negotiations: The concept of "principled negotiations"

Generally, the physician leader highly values relationships because they are the cornerstone of performance effectiveness. It has been pointed out by many observers that relationships play a major role in the conduct of negotiations. There is no question that one ordinarily negotiates much more forcefully when there is no current or future relationship between the two parties (for example, negotiating the purchase a car). However, the physician leader is very concerned about ongoing and future relationships in practically every negotiation. Nevertheless, that should not compromise your negotiating stance significantly if you utilize the concept of *principled negotiation*, as described by Ury and Fisher.[1] Principled negotiations include requirements that:

+ A *fair* agreement be reached that meets the interests of both parties.

+ The issues involved in the negotiations not be confused with the people who are negotiating.

+ The outcomes meet standards that are generally established and accepted by most people.

There is a very useful criterion for evaluating any negotiated agreement: Will the outcome, should it be revealed to others, bare the scrutiny of your peers? Sisela Bok, in her book *Lying: Moral Choice in Public and Private Life*, strongly promotes the notion of scrutiny by peers when evaluating the quality of your agreement.[2] Physician executives should make an absolute commitment to telling the truth when engaging in negotiations, although you need not disclose information that might place you at a disadvantage. One must assess carefully the difference between withholding information, at the risk of being deceptive, versus disclosing information that would weaken your negotiating posture. Because most negotiations conducted by physician leaders are part of a series, it is essential that you establish yourself as an individual who tells the truth and does not withhold information that should legitimately be disclosed.

If these rules are closely followed, there is little likelihood that relationships will suffer. In fact, relationships will likely prosper, because you will be perceived as a principled, fair individual who is able to find resolutions that have eluded others.

Know thyself

Just as a psychiatrist must intimately understand his own biases when conducting analysis, so must physician leaders intimately understand themselves. What is your most comfortable behavior? Are you hard-driving and competitive, or are you accommodating and primarily concerned with achieving good will? Are you bold and imaginative, or are you more comfortable with facts and figures, prone to careful analysis and favoring outcomes for which there is previous precedent? Do you try to persuade by using logic and rationale, or do you tend to be more assertive, to dominate and have a need "to win?" Perhaps you are idealistic and persuade by "inspiring" people to your point of view. Do you actively try to understand the other person's perspective, as reflected by engaging in questions such as "Do I understand you to say...? or "could I restate your argument as follows...?" In other words, are you a *good listener*? If not, you had better learn!

What does your body language say? Does it portray doubt and resistance, or does it encourage openmindedness? Is it overbearing or intimidating? Do you convey arrogance or condescension? Does it reflect sincere interest and concern? Your body language can be just as communicative as your verbal language in determining the outcome of a negotiation.

If you understand your biases, your behavior, and your body language, you are more likely to make the necessary adjustments in order to reach the desired outcome. Differences in language and style, as insightfully described by Deborah Tannen, are based on gender, ethnic background, social and economic class.[3] These differences frequently cause misunderstanding and a failure to communicate effectively.

Finally, choose your words carefully. Try to avoid words that have a pejorative or judgmental connotation. My involvement recently in an ethical consultation concerning the withdrawal of life support dramatically illustrated to me how individuals focus on a particular word. The son of the patient repeatedly focused on the use of the word "cruel." This word was used by the attending physician when discussing the futility of continuing to provide care to the mother, who was hopelessly and terminally ill. The son reacted defensively and resisted strongly any intimation that continuing to provide life support for his mother was "cruel." While I fully agreed with the attending physician's objective assessment, the choice of words in this case was detrimental to persuading the son to agree to withdraw life support for his terminally ill mother.

Another example is a mistake I made recently. In attempting to persuade radiologists at our hospital not to designate their contribution to the physicians' fund-raising campaign for radiology projects, I described the action as "self-serving" when viewed by others. The radiologists reacted negatively to this "accusation," focusing especially on the words "self-serving". I was not successful in my effort.

Know thy opponent

You should make every attempt to understand the individual with whom you are negotiating. Consider your opponent's biases, behavior, body language, and background in the same manner that you have tried to understand your own. What are that person's values? Are they economic, or do they reflect values of social justice? Is the person most interested in power, or do ethical issues have a higher priority? Are intellectual attainments, such as research or publications, driving the individual with whom you are negotiating? Values are primarily what motivate people to do the things they do, and your conceptual understanding of values is essential to understanding the art and science of negotiation. We tend to think of negotiations as being dominated by economic values, but other values often have a higher priority from the viewpoint of the person with whom you are negotiating. Not only should you understand your opposite's values, but you also need to get them on the table. What better way to find out than to ask openly, "What is really important to you?"

Information is critical. Every time you have information on what your opponent might want, you have more "currency" with which to negotiate. That is, you have discovered other "interests" that might be brought to the table and be offered as part of a negotiated agreement. A tug of war over financial positions, for example, can be resolved by providing other opportunities that are not financial but are, nevertheless, highly valued by your opposite. Such opportunities might include additional access, recognition by title, control of resources, etc. The admonition of Charles Dwyer is helpful to remember.[4] "Never expect anyone to engage in behavior that meets your needs unless you give them adequate reason to do so," i.e., behavior that they perceive as being in their best interests. Adequate reason can only be offered by thorough understanding of the issues, interests, values, and needs of the individual with whom you are negotiating.

The plan

It is most helpful to have a plan when you enter a negotiation. Such a plan is really no different than the system or outline that most physicians follow when obtaining a history. Many effective negotiators follow the concepts described by Ury and Fisher[1]:

Understand the issues as thoroughly as possible, and separate the issues from the people involved in the negotiation. The quickest way for a negotiation "to go South" is for the negotiators to attack the people involved rather than to concentrate on the issues attendant to the negotiation. Past history has to be discreetly put aside. Accusations attributed to motive, character, or past behavior will create friction and make a negotiation very difficult or, most likely, impossible. A thorough understanding and discussion of the issues will frequently reveal information that can be used later in the negotiation to achieve agreement. Moreover, the proper atmosphere for the negotiation is established as points of view are expressed and a good deal of listening is established. It is in this part of the negotiation that listening skills reflecting attention, questioning, understanding, and empathy are critical.

Discuss interests and not positions. How many times have you been involved in a disagreement and your adversary says, "My position is...." Consider that opening gambit. Does it not promote a certain obstinacy and rigidity? Frequently, the opening is followed by a long-winded rationalization and justification of the position. It is very difficult to have an effective meeting of the minds when this strategy is used. It places on the listener the obligation to state his or her "position" in equally strong terms and with equal justification. When a negotiation follows this path, the lines of battle are drawn, and the negotiators are usually far apart. Inordinate time is expended to bring the negotiating parties together.

Ury and Fisher suggest that negotiators concentrate on *interests* rather than on positions. Consider the following example of a recent negotiation conducted with our internists and cardiologists concerning the interpretation of ECGs on Medicare patients in the hospital. Recently, HCFA determined that it would not compensate physicians for professional interpretation of these ECGs. The interests of the cardiologists and internists were that they be reimbursed for the performance of a legitimate service at a reasonable amount. They also had an interest in not having the ECG interpretation put out to bid, either to a service outside the hospital or to a small group from within. The hospital's interests were that the ECGs continue to be interpreted by qualified individuals (a quality and safety interest), that it spend as little as possible (an economic interest of high priority because this represents incremental nonreimbursed expense for the hospital), and that it preserve its relationship with the internists and cardiologists (critically important for a hospital tightly engaged in competition). The expression of these interests by both parties to the negotiation resulted in a favorable agreement.

Imagine how different the results would have been if the internists and cardiologists had opened the negotiation with a statement of their "position": that the hospital should pay them x dollars to interpret ECGs on Medicare patients. Most likely, the hospital would have responded with a lower amount and a tug of war and bilateral threats would have begun. When there was clarification and understanding of mutual interests, agreement was much easier to achieve and both parties felt more fulfilled by the outcome.

45

The example above demonstrates that statement of positions frequently pre-empts discussion of interests. It places the outcome of the negotiation ahead of the discussion that should lead to the outcome. The importance of this discussion is not only to expose the interests of the negotiating parties, but also to provide the essential ingredient of participation in the process. Experienced negotiators will often tell you that the outcome of their negotiations was not very different from what they wanted prior to entering negotiations. Imagine how a participant would receive a resolution if appropriate discussion and participation had not occurred. A goal of principled negotiation is to get "buy in" of the agreement, and this only can be achieved through a participative process.

In summary, statement of positions draws lines of battle. Statement of interests opens doors for understanding and a sense of ownership of the agreement.

Consider alternative options. It is this stage of the negotiating process that often opens previously "locked doors." It is here that an imaginative and creative negotiator can be invaluable. Creative solutions are arrived at only when the negotiators thoroughly understand the values and interests of the parties to the negotiation. Ury and Fisher have described a useful list of needs that are common to most people:

✦ Security
✦ Economic well-being
✦ A sense of belonging
✦ Recognition
✦ Control of one's life or domain.

Why is it important to understand needs, and how do they open your imagination to alternative options for agreement? Superficially, many disputes confronting the physician leader appear to be economic in nature. For example, on behalf of the president of the medical staff, the Medical Executive Committee requests from administration an increase in salary from $15,000 to $30,000. The fact that the president is spending precious time on hospital affairs and could otherwise be earning money in his office is given as the ostensible reason. Consider the possible other options, using the concept of needs. Would recognition by the administration or the board of trustees be valuable in lieu of increased salary? Would a vote on the board of trustees give the medical staff a greater sense of participation and control of the decision making process? Would a longer term in office be valuable to the president? Would more staff support that would enable the president to be more efficient be a substitute for more salary? From administration's point of view, is this an opportunity to extract from the president more scheduled time with which to meet with the CEO or board committees? Would greater salary achieve more commitment from the president's partners to utilize the hospital rather than split patients with its competitor? Do the staff physicians achieve a greater sense of belonging because the president is being treated more respectfully? You may agree or disagree with any of these concepts as having relevance, but if you don't think about them or create others, you will continue to have tunnel vision regarding helpful options and alternatives.

To illustrate needs even more vividly, consider a dispute that the author witnessed between a radiology group and a group practice. The two parties were negotiating the salary for the radiologists who performed x-ray interpretations for films taken at the group practice location. On the surface, it appeared that the dispute was simply over money. However, it became obvious to me that, from the radiologists' perspective, the dispute had at least as much to do with recognition, belonging, and control as it did with financial remuneration. Repeatedly, the radiology negotiator complained that communication to him was conducted through a staff manager rather than a physician. The radiologists did not have input into the ordering or purchasing of equipment. They had no control over the transcription of reports and, because they were not allowed to have a key to the building, they frequently could not access the radiology suite to perform readings early in the morning or after the office had closed in the evening. Moreover, the radiologists much preferred to do their own professional billing rather than be salaried employees of the group practice. Had these issues of professional control been addressed, most certainly the outcome of the negotiation would not have been as protracted or nearly so bitter. Moreover, one can easily see that a number of different options and alternatives could have been introduced to the negotiation proceedings that would have considerably ameliorated the dispute over money and met the interests of both parties to the negotiation.

When considering options, it is essential to open your mind and not prejudge what initially appear to be hopeless and useless suggestions. It is a time for brainstorming and not critiquing. In fact, essential to the brainstorming process is that ideas are thrown on the table and not judged until later. Ury and Fisher use a circular chart[1] that emphasizes the description of the problem, the causes and symptoms of the problem, possible solutions that can be applied to fix the problem, and actions that can be taken to address the solution. In medical terms, this is analogous to the chief complaint and history, the physical exam, the diagnosis, and the treatment. Just as there frequently are many options and alternatives to treating a medical problem, there are numerous options and alternatives that can be applied to resolve disputes.

Apply reasonable standards to the negotiated agreement. It has been my observation that when a negotiated agreement reflects reasonable standards and objective criteria, it is generally a good one and is not likely to be broken. The agreement by the negotiators to apply such standards at the outset of negotiation immediately establishes the foundation for a principled agreement. If it appears early in negotiation that reasonable standards are not being requested by one of the parties, it becomes an effective strategy for the other party to indicate that he or she is going to insist upon reasonable standards and objective criteria.

Earlier in the chapter, it was mentioned that a principled agreement would bare the scrutiny of your peers. This is an effective litmus test for negotiated agreements and can be an internal standard frequently helpful as a guideline to your own flexibility in negotiations. While one would always attempt to maintain the confidentiality of agreements achieved through negotiation, one should also assume that information could become public. Agreements should never be a source of embarrassment to either party. As you negotiate, ask yourself, "How would this agreement be viewed by others should it become known?"

What kind of standards are appropriate to negotiated agreements in the context of health care? Agreements should be ethical. They should be legal. They should be within the norms of the industry and meet marketplace criteria. They should not establish precedents that you don't wish to repeat with others. They should be sensible in that they reflect legitimate pay for legitimate work. In summary, they should be fair and reflect common sense.

What if you cannot reach agreement?

Sometimes, despite your best efforts, you are not successful in achieving agreement. It is critical not to make a bad deal simply in the interests of resolution. A bad deal will always come home to haunt you sooner or later. If it doesn't haunt you, it is likely to haunt your successor!

Ury and Fisher have popularized the acronym BATNA, "best alternative to a negotiated agreement." The purpose of establishing a BATNA is that it forces you to consider your options ahead of time should you not be able to achieve an agreement. This exercise is critical, because it gives you negotiating confidence and forces you to examine a "worse case" scenario. That examination may well result in consideration of options and alternatives not previously examined. Failure to create a BATNA causes you to negotiate from weakness. You might make agreements that will not serve your best interests, and such agreements usually cause tremendous resentment at a later time. A BATNA differs from a "bottom line," which it sets limits but doesn't examine alternatives and options. To illustrate, let us consider the ECG negotiation referred to earlier in the chapter. The hospital could have established its BATNA as follows: if we cannot reach agreement at a reasonable level of reimbursement to the ECG readers, what will we do? Possible alternatives, each with advantages and disadvantages are to do nothing and allow each physician to interpret his or her own ECGs, have physicians obtain consultation to interpret ECGs, have the ECGs read by a computer and pay a cardiologist to "overread," put out for competitive bid ECG interpretation among groups within the hospital, or, finally, have an outside service read at a very low fee. One can see that simply by considering a BATNA, a whole host of alternative options are raised. Just considering these solutions allows you to internally evaluate the solution that you reach. One should be very suspicious of any agreement that is not as attractive as options created by reviewing your BATNA.

As in poker, you must know "when to hold and when to fold." When you fold in poker, you are out of that hand. However, you are not out of the game, and the next hand offers you new opportunities. Herb Cohen, author of *You Can Negotiate Anything*," puts it another way: "I care...but not that much."[5] If you "care too much" in a negotiation, the result will be the same as staying in a poker game with a poor hand.

If you cannot reach agreement in a negotiation, it is often useful to arrange for a third party to mediate. While one can formally request that an outside mediator be engaged, in health care organizations the third party mediator is frequently an individual who also has an interest in having the negotiation succeed. One can easily imagine that, in a dispute between two physicians, it is in the hospital's best interests to reach satisfactory resolution. In the example of the dispute between the medical group and the radiologists, it was clearly in the hospital's best interests to have the dispute favorably resolved. Indeed, when asked to assist in the resolution, the hospital was able to bring options to the table not previously available to the two negotiating parties. These options served the interests of all three parties.

Finally, consider the time-worn physician's axiom of "tincture of time." Frequently, a negotiation is not successfully concluded because the timing is not right. Generally, it is not advisable to be forced to conclude a negotiation because of time pressures. This is especially true when the time pressures are imposed by the other negotiating party. It is critical to evaluate the advantages and disadvantages of delay against those of quick closure. For example, consider your decision to buy a house. Are you getting the best price now, or will prices go down over the next few months? Will the house still be available if you wait? What alternatives will be available if waiting causes you to lose this house? Will mortgage rates rise or fall in the near future? Is this the house that you really want, or are you willing to consider other locations, styles, sizes, price ranges, distance from work, etc? With the passage of time, change occurs. Evaluate the consequences of change carefully when negotiating.

Summary

In this chapter, I have emphasized the importance of negotiation skills for the new physician leader. While relationships are vital to your success, one should discard the notion that being a good negotiator places relationships at risk. The concept of principled negotiation has been advanced to enhance the power of the physician leader; create new, unimagined opportunities; as well as minimize the risk of disturbing relationships. Moreover, no individual in the organization is better suited to engage in negotiations involving physicians than you, the new physician leader.

It is very important for you to understand yourself in terms of your behavior, your language, and your body language. What messages are you sending, consciously or unconsciously? Likewise, it is equally important that you understand your counterpart and "read between the lines." What is he or she really saying? Values that motivate people and common needs that require satisfaction have been discussed in the context of understanding alternative viewpoints and facilitating new options for agreement.

The concepts of principled negotiation have been elucidated: separate the people from the issues, discuss interests and not positions, examine many alternatives and options, and reach agreements that reflect acceptable standards and criteria. In addition, it has been strongly suggested that any agreement pass the test of "scrutiny by your peers." Principles of truth-telling and fairness are fundamental to favorable, durable agreements. A systematized approach, using a negotiating plan, is recommended when entering a negotiation. The analogy has been made to the physician's systematized approach to performing a history and physical exam.

Finally, if all avenues are exhausted and agreement cannot be achieved, the strategy of the BATNA (best alternative to a negotiated agreement) is recommended. Advantages of bringing in a third party to the negotiation should be evaluated, as well as the options of mediation or arbitration. Resorting to legal action has not been discussed, as it generally reflects a failure of the negotiation process.

References

1. Ury, W., and Fisher, R. *Getting to Yes*. Boston, Mass.: Houghton-Mifflin, 1981.

2. Bok, S. *Lying: Moral Choice in Public and Private Life*. New York, N.Y.: Random House, 1979.

3. Tannen, D. *You Just Don't Understand*. New York, N.Y.: William Morrow & Company, 1990.

4. Dwyer, C. *The Shifting Sources of Power and Influence*. Tampa, Fla.: American College of Physician Executives, 1992.

5. Cohen, H. *You Can Negotiate Anything*. New York, N.Y.: Bantam Books, 1982.

Howard E. Rotner, MD, FACPE, is Medical Director, AtlantiCare Medical Center, Lynn, Massachusetts.

CHAPTER 6

Conflict Management

by James M. Richardson, MD, FACP, FACPE

*C*ommunication is the essential ingredient that allows people to relate to one another. It is essential on both personal and business levels. When effective communications fails, one of the things that often occurs is conflict. The conflict may be a simple disagreement in regard to ideas, issues, or interests, or it may be more complex, extreme, and destructive. The latter case of communication failure is called dysfunctional conflict. It is never desirable or necessary. It is always bad, even at its best. Managers cannot afford to have dysfunctional conflict in their organizations, but unless they manage conflict by being effective communicators, recognizing situations that will convert simple conflict into more complex conflict, dysfunctional conflict will be inevitable. The principles discussed in this chapter apply to any persons or groups involved in personal or business relationships.

Simple Conflict

Conflict is a naturally occurring phenomenon. It is to be expected in individual or group situations. The need to deal with conflict resolution is a common and time-consuming process. Being able to effectively deal with conflict episodes depends on how well the manager understands the dynamics and how well he or she can identify the features on which intervention can occur.

Effective conflict management requires skills that have to be learned. The skills required are in oral, written, and nonverbal communications; in preventing, recognizing, and removing the barriers to communication; and in active listening and feedback.

Conflict is a subjective phenomenon. Depending on how it is perceived in the minds of the individuals involved, it becomes objective only in the sense that its manifestations are real, through the acting out, the anger, the attacks, etc. Because conflict is subjective, it is emotional. One can, therefore, understand how, during conflict episodes, basic communication is impaired, reasoning and perceptions are distorted, attacks become personal, and the overall situation tends to deteriorate.

It is easy to automatically consider conflict to be negative. When this occurs, the consequences are predictably adverse. If conflict is viewed as being a positive force, a completely different outcome is possible. With this latter view of conflict, a process can be initiated that can result in full identification of problems, understanding of the points of view of others, evaluation of alternatives, stimulation of interest, involvement of people in such a way that they will become committed, and willingness to devote the energy necessary for implementation of a successful project. In other words, the positive consequences of conflict can include the evolution of new or modified goals, closer interpersonal relationships, effective problem-solving, and end-results that are far superior to those originally envisioned.

Dysfunctional Conflict

Dysfunctional conflict is a negative force. It occurs at a high price. Not only do emotions run high, but anger and hostility are exhibited; the primary problem or issue becomes subverted; stress is created; efficiency, effectiveness, and productivity are lowered; there is damage to interpersonal relationships, with respect and trust being lost, at least for the short term; and time, energy, and money are wasted.

In order for conflict to occur and develop, there must be an underlying cause or condition of which both parties are aware. The involved parties respond to the condition with feelings of tension, irritation, actions, and counteractions. Finally, the end defines the type of result that comes from the conflict episode. Was it satisfactorily or unsatisfactorily settled? Were the issues in the conflict resolved? If not resolved, the conflict episode is sure to recur.

Causes of Conflict

There are six major causes of conflict in organizations:

✦ Basic failure in communication, including a misconception of information—Just as effective communication can affect the organization's efficiency and effectiveness and the quality of its products or services, a failure to communicate effectively can cause organizational conflict.

✦ The threat of change—Because everything is in a state of change, change is inevitable, and no change is final. Change involves the future and the future is unknown. We fear the unknown. When the unknown involves us personally and adversely, we feel insecure. This insecurity provokes in us a negative action that is manifested in an emotional way. This action further provokes a spiraling series of counteractions. Each person responds differently to the stresses caused by change, making for different outcomes, which are unpredictable.

The results of change have differing impacts, depending on whether there are external or internal forces affecting the organization. External forces often are in the form of constraints. They may include changes in laws, regulations, funding, competition, etc. They can affect the individual, but they are more likely to have a direct impact on the organization and its resources. Internal forces are more likely to affect the power structure or organizational arrangement. Issues of authority, power, control, position, economics, and security come into play.

In an organization, change can best be dealt with in a systematic fashion. At the time of an anticipated significant change, there needs to be a determination of the scope of the problems that will develop as a result of the change. This cannot or usually should not be done by the manager alone. In addition, neither should the development, analysis, and selection of alternatives or the implementation and evaluation of the change be the responsibilities of the manager alone. With the participative style of management, the goal is to have appropriate staff involvement. With commitment, there is acceptance of decisions made, and, with acceptance, there is the required energy and time necessary to make it possible for decisions to be successfully implemented. These are advantages over the autocratic style of management, which institutes change independently by oral or written communication.

✦ Competition for limited resources—Resources are always limited. In most organizations, critical limitations of resource allocation are a frequent reason for competition between individuals, groups, or departments and are a source of conflict. The resource may be money, space, equipment, computer time, etc.

✦ Differences regarding organizational goals—Such differences are a frequent cause of organizational conflict. The differences occur in spite of the fact that it is clear to most employees that top management or the board of directors determines the mission of the organization and sets the organization's policies and goals. It is the responsibility of middle management, through strategic planning and with top management's approval, to establish departmental goals and objectives by which organizational goals can be achieved. It is lower level management's responsibility to develop procedures to achieve day-to-day goals and objectives that will produce products or services. In spite of the best efforts, differences occur in the perception of the overall goals, priorities, methods, resource utilization, etc. When these ideas are the same, there is no conflict.

✦ Ambiguities in organizational structure—The structure of the organization may be poor, allowing for overlapping responsibilities, gaps in responsibilities, and inconsistent and conflicting policies.

✦ Differences regarding performance standards and expectations—Although performance standards and expectations initially affect individuals and can cause conflicts, they eventually affect the entire organization and the products or services that are to be delivered.

Avoiding Conflict

Before delineating specific ways to avoid conflict in organizations, two characteristics of vital importance must be discussed. They are frequently underemphasized, and involve, (a) shared values, and (b) having trust in the person(s) or group with whom you are dealing.

Organizational Values

Just as values and value systems are important to individuals, they are also important to organizations. Values represent the desirability or worth of a thing; they are a moral precept. The organization's value system not only influences its ethical standards, but also is the foundation for its code of ethics. It influences staff behavior. The value system determines how hard and how long a person will fight for something. Values are very hard to change. When our values are threatened, our integrity is threatened. But values are just an abstraction until choices have to be made. Hard decisions are value judgments. The quality of an organization's value system is seen in the types of hard decisions it makes. An organization's budget also is representative of its values.

Because personal and organizational values are so basic, if one party knows the other party's values, the behavior and decisions of the other party can be, to some degree, predicted. In decision making, the individual or organization should determine the value of a significant point at issue and then make the decision. This is value-based decision making. It can make decision making easier, especially if there is no incongruence between values and the actions taken. And as expected, core values make up the organization's mission statement. It is differences in values that are often the sources of conflict.

Trust

Good interpersonal relationships are essential to any effective communications process, and fundamental to good interpersonal relationships is the need for trust between individuals and groups. Trust is a feeling of being safe, confident, accepted, respected, reliant, consistent, and devoid of fear, even in the presence of disagreement. Trust is a subjective feeling. Being trustworthy is based on a summation of things—what we say, how we say it, what we do, how we do it, honesty, integrity, our behavior, actions, responses, sensitivity, empathy, etc. We cannot set as an objective the creation of a sense of trustworthiness. Being trustworthy comes from an inner quality and strength, namely, good ethical and moral character, the absence of which cannot be covered up for long.

Personal Issues

Also of great importance in avoiding conflict is to keep issues nonpersonalized, which means to avoid focusing on principles, morals, religious beliefs, or ethical issues. Once any one of these four issues is raised, it usually becomes a win/lose situation. We naturally tend to defend our self-image and issues of principle, morals, religion, and ethics uncompromisingly. "Losing face" or sacrificing integrity is at stake. An impasse in conflict resolution usually results. Sometimes the only way to get beyond this impasse is for both parties to agree to disagree.

Other Ways To Avoid Conflict

Other ways to avoid conflict in management are:

✦ Remain calm.
✦ Disarm the other party by not responding as he or she does.
✦ Disclose something that will be interpreted as a positive move.
✦ Avoid statements that begin with "you."
✦ Avoid accusations such as "you always" or "you never."
✦ Avoid the "no" word.
✦ Avoid judgmental statements such as "Why did you do that?"
✦ Avoid insults to the other party's ego.
✦ Avoid words or actions that will escalate the conflict episode.

Beginning Conflict Resolution

The purpose of the process of conflict resolution is to:

✦ Present thoughtful alternatives so that conflict will be converted into collaboration.
✦ Validate the values of the other party.
✦ Appear fair.
✦ Accept some responsibility.
✦ Promote a spirit of understanding and cooperation.
✦ Look for opportunities to improve interpersonal relationships.

Perceived Differences

If there is a significant perceived difference in strength, authority, or technical advantage in either party's favor, the resolution process is likely to be more difficult. This situation can exist between manager and subordinate, manager and colleague, or management and union representatives. The difficulty may be that the stronger party may be more likely to want to impose a solution or that the weaker party, because of his or her situation, may have to accept a solution that is far from satisfactory.

Managers, by their very positions, have authority and power. How much authority and power there is depends on many factors. One's authority will depend on the job description, but, just as important, it depends on how the person in the position executes authority. The person may gain or give up authority that is inherent in the job.

Power can be considered the perception of others about how well someone can influence or effect change, about the person's ability to exercise control. Because authority and power are necessary for managers in their decision making, it is only a matter of time before managers generate conflict. This is because managerial decisions will eventually restrict the autonomy of some colleagues and subordinates. It is therefore essential for managers to use their abilities, authority, and power to the utmost in managing conflict in order to minimize the possibility that dysfunctional conflict will develop.

Unreadiness
The two parties involved in a conflict episode must perceive that a conflict exists, but, before they are ready to resolve the conflict, there is an escalation phase when resolution is impossible. This is the period when accusations, insults, hostility, and anger are prevalent. It is not until at least one of the parties wants to seek a resolution to the conflict that there can be attempts at successful conflict resolution.

Confrontation
In addition, there has to be confrontation during a conflict episode if there is to be conflict resolution. Otherwise compromise, postponement, or avoidance will usually occur. The word "confrontation," from one aspect, is similar to the word "conflict." It can and should be looked at in terms of possible positive consequences. Confrontation in regard to issues in conflict can and should result in an improved outcome. If the conflict worsens and dysfunctional conflict occurs, the process has failed.

Confrontation in conflict resolution usually involves six major steps, according to Newstrom and Davis.[1]

+ Awareness—There is recognition by at least one person or group involved that a conflict exists, and they are willing to initiate the confrontation.

+ Confrontation is decided—Both persons or groups decide that the issue is important enough not to be avoided and that confrontation will resolve the differences.

+ Confrontation occurs—The response of the opposing persons or groups will determine if there is acceptance of the confrontation, denial, a reduction in the seriousness of the conflict, escalation, or resolution of the conflict.

+ Determination of the cause of the conflict—At this step, if the issue is focused and the opposing parties share information and describe their opinions and feelings, the cause for the conflict can be determined.

+ Development of solutions—Here, the opposing parties work toward eliminating or reducing the causes of the conflict.

+ Follow-up—For long-term success of the solution, both parties must make regular checks to verify that agreements are being kept.

When this process has been successful, the positive aspects of conflict episodes are exemplified because the two parties have worked together to solve problems.

Strategies in Conflict Resolution

If conflict is to be resolved satisfactorily, it must be approached and dealt with correctly. An unsatisfactory strategy will most likely result in an unsatisfactory outcome. The strategy can be goal-directed (what benefits both parties) or outcome-directed (who gets what). Filley's studies describe three forms of conflict strategies—win/lose, lose/lose, and win/win.[2] These are the same strategies recommended for formal and informal negotiations.

Possible Outcomes

The strategy selected will determine if the conflict episode will be:

+ Positive or negative.
+ Personalized or objective.
+ Goals or outcome directed.
+ Victory or defeat.
+ Satisfactory or unsatisfactory.
+ Resolved or unresolved.
+ Finished or recurring.

Win/Lose

Individuals as well as departments within organizations often oppose one another in order to gain prestige, power, or resources or to show dominance. If the win/lose strategy is selected, one party will be the winner, the other the loser. The loser will likely be angry and hostile and will not be a fully committed and involved participant in the implementation of solutions. The winner is, therefore, not a true winner, because friendship and future cooperation by the other party may be lost. It is noteworthy that the practice of voting in these circumstances formalizes the win/lose strategy and should be avoided.

Lose/Lose

Just as the lose/lose strategy suggests, neither party wins, the conflict is not resolved, and a solution is not reached, even though each party may have gained something.

Win/Win

The win/win strategy to resolve conflict is most desirable. The solution is agreed upon and is satisfactory to both parties, even though neither party may have received all of what it initially sought. The parties commit to implementation of the solution and involve themselves with the energy necessary to achieve success.

The win/win strategy usually results in solutions by consensus or by integration. When this happens, alternatives have been thoroughly examined. True consensus is ideal, but usually takes a long time, requires a lot of energy, and is difficult to achieve. The larger the opposing parties, the greater the difficulty. When consensus occurs, the focus is on problem solving, not the solution itself.

The Integrative Approach

When the integrative approach is used, goals and values, not solutions, are stressed. Filley describes several characteristics necessary for the integrative approach[2]:

+ Clearly defined issues.
+ A focus on goals and objectives.
+ A genuine search for alternatives.
+ A lack of time constraints.
+ A truly interactive process.
+ The sharing of information.
+ Open mindedness.
+ Leadership that is flexible.
+ Trust.
+ Acceptance of solutions.

Third-Party Intervention

When a conflict episode has resulted in a win/lose confrontation, a third party may have to intercede through mediation or arbitration. Facts alone and attempts at persuasion are usually ineffective. In this situation, a change in attitude or position is necessary if there is to be movement toward resolution of the issues.

The mediator should be neutral, prestigious, trusted, and respected by both parties. He or she can provide the forum for new information to be shared, for the feelings of the opposite person or group to be known, for reasonable and constructive stances to be taken, and, ultimately, for there to be a change of attitude or position.

Mediation is preferable to arbitration, because arbitration is usually judgmental and often results in a win/lose or lose/lose conclusion. Mediation provides the opportunity for true conflict resolution and a win/win conclusion.

Conflict Resolution in Large Groups

The process for conflict resolution in large groups can be quite different from dealing with a small number of individuals. The mediator usually meets independently and dually with representatives of each group and, according to Newstrom and Davis,[1] often functions in the following manner:

+ Prepares—Before the opposing groups meet, the mediator prepares them for meeting one another, in part by encouraging an approach that is positive, open-minded, frank, and constructive.

+ Controls discussion—The mediator controls the content and the pace of meetings and maintains the peace.

+ Permits role reversal—Each side learns to understand the position of the opposition.

✦ Defuses tension—The mediator facilitates the expression of feelings, including anger and frustration, in a constructive manner.

✦ Transmits information—Information is given to each side to facilitate the communication process.

✦ Formulates proposals—At the appropriate time, possible solutions are suggested by the mediator.

Methods for Implementing Strategy

After a satisfactory conflict-reducing strategy is developed, implementation of the strategy is necessary. According to Blake et al., this step can involve five methods[3]:

✦ Compromising—This is a process of problem solving using mutual concession.

✦ Confronting or Problem Solving—Facing the problem head on, rather than avoiding it. The cause for conflict is identified and eliminated during this process.

✦ Forcing—This method uses physical, intellectual, ethical, and moral pressures.

✦ Smoothing—Decreasing the harshness, crudeness, unpleasantness, and distasteful component of the conflict episode is attempted.

✦ Withdrawing—This involves withdrawing, retreating, or disengaging from the conflict.

Confronting and smoothing result in constructive handling of the situation. Withdrawing and forcing result in adverse outcomes. The impact of compromising is relatively neutral in regard to reducing conflict.

Other Components of Strategy

There are other components of strategy that are necessary for successful conflict resolution:

✦ Preparation—This is achieved through learning a wide variety of interpersonal communication skills, understanding the dynamics of organizational conflict, managing change and the resistance to it, overcoming dysfunctional individual and group behavior, and keeping dialogue open and frank.

✦ Early intervention.

✦ Keeping issues focused.

✦ Depersonalization of the problem—When a problem becomes personalized, all the dynamics of defensiveness come into play, resulting in intensification of the seriousness of the problem. When the focus is on persons or personalities, the conflict is sure to continue.

Know the Other Party

It is essential to know the other parties with whom you are dealing. Learn their values, personalities, emotional makeup, likes, and dislikes. If the parties involved in a conflict have worked together successfully in the past and will have to work together in the future, they are more likely to approach the situation from a win/win perspective. On the contrary, if this is a first encounter and they are not likely to be involved in future relationships, a win-lose perspective will more likely be followed. The conflict will be more difficult to resolve, and, at the conclusion, one party will be dissatisfied.

Cooling Off

Early on in the conflict episode, there may be the need for a cooling off period in order for there to be calm, reasoned, and rational discussion. The length of the cooling off period (minutes, hours, or days) will depend on a number of factors:

+ The seriousness and duration of the conflict.

+ How hardened opposing views are.

+ The level of the emotional state or tension.

+ Past experience the opposing parties have had in dealing with one another and the success of those experiences.

+ How they feel about one another at the time of the current conflict episode.

Summary

Conflict in organizations is inevitable, but every effort should be made to prevent dysfunctional conflict and its costly consequences. Prevention is possible only if the manager develops good interpersonal relationships, learns effective communication skills, and recognizes and manages conflict episodes when they first begin.

References

1. Newstrom, J., and Davis, K. *Organizational Behavior.* New York, N.Y.: McGraw-Hill Book Co., 1989.

2. Filley, A. *"Conflict Resolution: The Ethic of the Good Loser"* in Huseman, R., et al., Eds., Readings in Interpersonal and Organizational Communication, 3rd Edition. Boston, Mass.: Holbrook Press, 1977.

3. Blake, R., and others. *Managing Intergroup: Conflict in Industry.* Houston, Tex.: Gulf Publishing, 1964.

Further Reading

Dubrin, A. *Fundamentals of Organizational Behavior—An Applied Perspective.* Elmsford, N.Y.: Pergamon, 1974, p. 312.

Huseman, R., and others. *"Interpersonal Conflict in the Modern Organization"* in Readings in Interpersonal and Organizational Communication, 3rd Edition, Boston, Mass.: Holbrook Press, 1977.

Keating, C. *Dealing with Difficult People—How You Can Come out on Top in Personality Conflicts.* New York, N.Y.: Paulist Press, 1984.

Montana, P., and Charnov, B. *Barron's Business Review Series.* New York, N.Y.: Barron's, 1987, p. 300-29.

Pondy, L. *"Organizational Conflict: Concepts and Models."* Administrative Science Quarterly 12(9):299-306, Sept. 1967.

Rasberry, R., and Lemoine, L. *Effective Managerial Communication.* Boston, Mass.: Kent Publishing Co., 1986. p. 377-94.

Richardson, J. "Communicator, Know Thyself." *Physician Executive* 14(3):19-21, May-June 1988.

Richardson, J. "Defensive Barriers to Communications." *Physician Executive* 16(5):37-8, Sept.-Oct. 1990.

Richardson, J. "Management of Conflict in Organizations." *Physician Executive* 17(1):39-42, Jan.-Feb. 1991.

Richardson, J. "Listening and Feedback: Two Essentials for Interpersonal Communication." *Physician Executive* 17(2)35-8, March-April 1991.

Selye, H. *Stress without Distress.* New York, N.Y.: New American Library, 1975.

James M. Richardson, MD, FACP, FACPE, is Medical Director, Fairmont Hospital, San Leandro, Calif., and an Assistant Clinical Professor of Medicine, University of California, San Francisco. He is a Distinguished Fellow of the American College of Physician Executives and a Fellow of the American College of Physicians.

CHAPTER 7

Organizational Politics

by Robert A. Kramer, MD

*P*olitics is defined as the "art or science of government" or "the art or science concerned with guiding or influencing governmental policy." Skill in organizational politics implies a thorough knowledge of the rules of governance within the organization—how to influence their interpretation and how to apply them. The physician who becomes part of an organization, particularly as a department head, ignores these rules at his or her own peril. The rules of an organization exist in two major forms. The formal rules appear in the bylaws and the rules and regulations. The informal rules are the customs or corporate culture of the organization, which are rarely documented but must be fully understood in order to be an effective player. Another key guide to organizational politics is the table of organization, which purports to describe the reporting relationships within the organization. As with the unwritten rules, there will be relationships that do not strictly conform to the table of organization. Such relationships evolve either from previous connections of the parties or within the context of their responsibilities. The table of organization may also be distorted by the strength or weakness of any given individual within the structure.

The pitfalls for the clinical department chief evolve from misunderstanding the organization's explicit or implicit rules and the written and unwritten relationships in the table of organization. The first steps in learning an organization's politics are understanding one's own position description; the true level of responsibility assigned to the position; the reporting hierarchy; and the sources of power of the position. It is not sufficient to have the bylaws and the table of organization. Perceptions of the clinical department chief's position by all those to whom the position reports, and by all those who report to the position are often more important than written expectations.

This chapter will describe some of the typical organizational pitfalls for the clinical department chief and some strategies to overcome them. The objective is to be able to anticipate problems and apply preventive methods to them. A typical table of organization is shown in the figure below. It is very important that the clinical department chief understand who are his or her organizational peers and who is placed at a reporting level above him or her. Many of the organizational pitfalls to which a newly appointed clinical department chief must be sensitive lie within this structure.

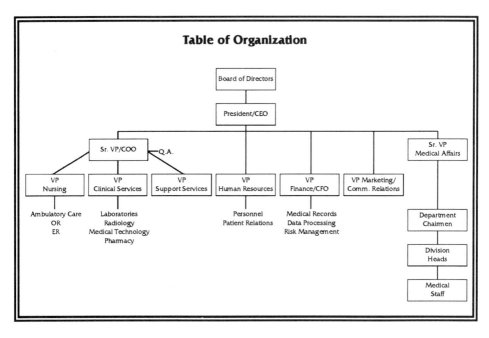

Pitfall #1—Misunderstanding one's location in the table of organization.

It is very easy to make assumptions as one enters into this position in respect to one's relationships with other individuals in the table of organization. This is particularly sensitive when the new clinical department chief has come from the attending staff of the hospital. As a private practice attending, the physician feels no relationship to the table of organization. It is not unusual for a senior attending to be at ease with and on a first name relationship with members of the board, the CEO, the president of the medical staff, the vice president of medical affairs, and the vice president of nursing, as well as many of the department heads of the hospital. To assume that the relationship will be the same with each of these individuals when one becomes a salaried member of the organization and is subject to organizational politics and/or rules can guarantee conflict. Not only do individuals higher up on the table of organization expect recognition of their positions; they also become very sensitive about approaches that don't go through channels and don't take cognizance of reporting relationships.

Strategy: The clinical department chief must have a clear understanding of the differences between the individual entrepreneur and the organizational person. It is imperative that the relationships and the expectations of the various members of the organization toward this position be clearly spelled out and accepted before making a commitment to becoming a member of the organization. Interviews with principals in the organization to determine their expectations of the clinical chief's relationships are invaluable.

Pitfall #2—Taking advantage of long-established social or professional relationships with board members or senior administrators, bypassing the vice president for medical affairs and/or the CEO.

It is natural to take advantage of established relationships with the sincere intent of expediting a project. The risk is in bypassing individuals to whom the clinical chief reports and who themselves may have a reporting relationship with those in the chief's old network. This can set up serious resentments and can be perceived as evidence of lack of commitment to the organization or, even worse, disloyalty and ignorance of procedure.

Strategy: No matter how easy or tempting the communication may be, all discussions with board or administrative friends relevant to the professional function of the clinical department chief or the institution itself should be made known to the medical director or vice president for medical affairs or to whomever the clinical department chief reports. Be prepared to delay or reconsider the communication if it conflicts with the goals and objectives of the medical director. A successful executive becomes a student of the style, as well as the goals and objectives, of his or her boss. The clinical chief must consistently reinforce in the mind of the vice president for medical affairs or medical director that he or she is loyal; capable of receiving or giving honest criticism; and, above all, prepared to recommend solutions to problems that are identified.

It is reasonable to expect the CEO to want to have a close relationship with the clinical department chiefs of a hospital. The CEO may perceive this level of management as critical to the success of the organization and may even bypass the vice president for medical affairs in his or her outreach to the clinical department chiefs. As welcome as such communications may be, it is in the best interests of the clinical department chief and the organization that the clinical chief keep the dialogue inclusive of the vice president for medical affairs, particularly when it has to do with access to resources or program development within the hospital.

Pitfall #3—Approaching the vice president for nursing as a peer or, even worse, as being in a subservient position.

In virtually all hospitals today, the vice president for nursing ranks on at least the same level as other vice presidents reporting to the chief executive officer and is not perceived by the rest of the organization or by the vice president for nursing as a peer of clinical department chiefs. It is probable that the vice president for nursing is even more sensitive to organizational politics than most clinical department chiefs may be. The vice president for nursing generally commands the largest group of professionals in the hospital and can be expected to be their advocate and protector.

Strategy: Winning the respect and receptivity of the vice president for nursing is critical for the success of the clinical department chief. A sense of partnership can be communicated, along with clear respect for the position and the power that has been invested in the vice president of nursing. The nursing profession has become exquisitely sensitive to reporting relationships and expects clinical department chiefs to be equally sensitive. It is also important to remember that many nursing executives recall the experience of being treated as a servant by the physician and will have their antennae extended to detect any evidence of the classical physician superiority over nursing. Again, recognize that most training programs for nursing executives include considerable emphasis on the organization and the relationships within it. By the same token, the classical partnership of physician and nurse on behalf of the patient can still be effectively used in this context.

Other individuals on the vice president level to whom the clinical department chief similarly may relate include vice presidents for clinical affairs and support services, who may be responsible for the resources that the clinical department head must obtain, be it equipment, personnel, space or financial support. The professionals at the vice president level can be expected to be well-trained in their respective areas of responsibility and to be totally committed to the welfare of the institution and more loyal to the chief executive officer than to the department head. Any approach to them that does not recognize their responsibility or their relationships to other clinical department chiefs could lead to loss of both the objective and future receptivity. The clinical chief must get to know the interests and perceptions of the roles of each of the individuals on the vice president level. It is imperative to demonstrate understanding and respect for their positions.

Pitfall #4—Treating the chief financial officer as just another "bean counter."

In today's world of tight regulation, governmental oversight, and third-party payer review, the chief financial officer is called upon by the administration and the board of the hospital not only to account for its finances, but also to protect the hospital from financial risks, both internal and external. The CEO of the hospital can be expected to have a very close relationship with the chief financial officer, and the chief financial officer can be expected to have substantial influence on both the CEO and the board. The role of the chief financial officer in program review is to stress fiscal responsibility, not clinical efficacy.

Strategy: With the blessing of the vice president for medical affairs, the clinical department chief can seek understanding of the chief financial officer's perceptions of his department's contribution to the hospital, as well as its needs for resources. Most CFOs will be very supportive of a department where they see creative initiatives to improve the bottom line. They will understand the importance of a department that supports the hospital's mission but is not producing a positive balance. Recognizing the culture of the institution, it is important to be sure that these messages are transmitted to the CFO through the vice president for medical affairs or with his concurrence. It is likely that the CFO will be a major participant in the review of new programs submitted by a department chief, as well as the assessment of the effectiveness of existing programs. It is the CFO's job to challenge the value of any program to the financial health of the institution. If the CFO perceives the department chief as a thoughtful and conscientious manager who is concerned about revenue and expenses, he or she is more likely to give an objective review of the department's programs. Where a department is not able to produce a positive balance, the CFO will seek evidence that the clinical chief is managing resources with maximum efficiency.

Pitfall #5—Unfair or unnecessary competition with other clinical department chiefs.

As illustrated by the table of organization, other clinical department chiefs are peers within the organization. Each department chief can be expected to strive for a fair share of hospital resources. However, there will be those whose departments contribute more to the financial health of the institution and others whose contribution cannot be measured in terms of revenue production. Traditionally medical and surgical specialties that generate substantial revenue to the hospital have more power than departments that do not. However, the assumption that the dollar contribution of any given clinical department chief's staff guarantees that department's preferential access to resources or control within the institution cannot and should not be taken for granted. The problem lies in the perspective or management style of the vice president for medical affairs, the chief financial officer, and the president and CEO of the hospital. In the absence of a balanced and even-handed approach to access to resources or control, there may be individual chiefs who exceed authority, ignore institutional guidelines, or exert undeserving influence on the management process.

Strategy: The clinical department chief needs to establish a clear understanding with members of his or her peer group as to their contribution to the health of the institution, both financially and professionally, and establish both credibility and interdependence among the clinical chiefs. The clinical chief should seek evidence of an institutional commitment to effective partnership and collaboration among clinical department chiefs. It is important that there be peer-level loyalty, as well as respect for the goals and objectives of the institution itself. It is imperative that the clinical chief be empowered to negotiate for resources among fellow clinical chiefs and that the chiefs be mutually supportive in their requests for hospital resources. Because very few hospitals have unlimited access to such resources, department chiefs need to have assurances that their requests will be given a fair hearing by the administration and that there is a hospital-sanctioned method for appealing decisions when there are conflicting objectives. The new department chief should have a clear understanding of the options in this area. The clinical chief should also have an understanding of the role of the vice president for medical affairs in conflict resolution among the department chiefs.

Pitfall #6—Trying to retain the same collegial relationship with medical practitioners that existed before the role of department chief was assumed.

It is the nature of physicians moving from the clinical realm to the administrative role to try to hold on to relationships and the image of the practicing physician, even though there is a genuine commitment to administrative/management responsibility. The challenge of making decisions that affect the ability of a former colleague to practice; to have specific privileges within the hospital; and/or to be compensated for his or her professional efforts places a significant strain on previous relationships. These responsibilities require a redefinition of relationships with medical peers.

Strategy: With the help of the vice president for medical affairs or the medical director, the areas of responsibility and control for the clinical department chief needs to be communicated to division chiefs and to medical staff members within the chief's department. For the newly arrived chief, it is appropriate to know whether department members participated in defining the role of the chief or whether the decision was made at a higher level and thrust upon them. Depending on which style of management was used, the new chief needs to meet with department members and establish their expectations of the department chief. It is then appropriate to give department members a clear understanding of the expectations of the chief—what the chief's goals and objectives are for the department as well as expectations for the department's relationship with the institution—and some insight as to the new chief's administrative style. This is achieved through open meetings with the staff. In some circumstances, meetings with the staff prior to commitment to the appointment can establish relationships and understandings that will be invaluable once the new chief is in place. There needs to be a thorough understanding of institutional management style and culture before seeking this type of introduction. In the case of the chief who has been recruited from among the practicing attendings in the department, one must provide colleagues with an opportunity to define the impact of the new position on their past relationships—how will they have access to the chief and how much can old obligations be called upon in this new relationship. It is important to be sure that all staff members understand and respect the change in relationships.

Pitfall #7—Ignorance of the history of the institution.

As important as it is to know the corporate culture of the hospital, it is equally important to know the history of the institution. It is important to know the timing of the major events in the institution's history from its very origins. It is equally important to know about the organization or individuals that brought the institution into existence. The history of the physical plant and the timing of the addition of major services to the institution are a useful part of one's background knowledge as well. The political forces in the community among sister institutions, government, and other organizations is important to understand, particularly as one looks at the long-range plans and mission of the hospital.

Within the history may lie the story of struggles for primacy of any given department or program; conflicts of predecessors with other departments, management, or the board; clinical or management failures; clinical or management successes; and a chain of relationships that may be important to understand in negotiating the political corridors of the institution. It is important to know who is revered and who is feared in the institution's history. The reputation of the institution among the professional and lay community is particularly important to understand for the newcomer to the community. Other valuable bits of history would include the rate of turnover of management positions on the medical-administrative staff; the tenure of one's predecessor and his or her reasons for leaving; and, as best one can determine, whatever "baggage" comes with the position.

Strategy: Clearly, it is in the best interests of the new clinical chief to learn as much of the chronological and political history of the hospital and the department as is available. This may exist in both written documents and oral history. Senior members of the department or the institution or community leaders can provide a historical narrative of the growth and development of the department and the institution and should be sought out before making a commitment to the position. Among important historical data that should be examined is the history of benefactors to the department and the results of external evaluations that may have been commissioned.

Pitfall #8—Impatience with the process.

Inertia is characteristic of large organizations. As the complexity of the organization expands and the number of individuals who must be involved in decision making increases, the degree of inertia increases. This is particularly an issue for the clinical chief who comes from the private practice of medicine. In that setting, the expectation that one's wishes become one's commands and that one's staff responds promptly to such wishes can no longer be the case. Although impatience may be tactfully applied, if it becomes a characteristic response to institutional inertia, the clinical chief can become labeled and lose both credibility and sympathy.

Strategy: A clinical chief can demonstrate his or her impatience with process as long as there is evidence that the demonstration of impatience is restricted to clinical imperatives where patients are put at risk and does not represent a generic reaction to all procedures. The clinical chief will be respected by the administrative hierarchy when the impatience is so applied and when there is evidence that it is applied with restraint and clear justification. Again, it is very important for the clinical chief to avoid the perception of responding to all processes with impatience. This will only result in loss of credibility.

Pitfall #9—Mismanaging one's mistakes.

No one can assume a management role without the risk of error. The error can only be compounded if it is not properly recognized, acknowledged and corrected.

Any attempt to avoid confrontation with one's errors or to cover them up will be detrimental to one's effectiveness as a manager or a leader. The process by which mistakes are identified and addressed should be understood and communicated to both peers and those to whom the chief reports.

Strategy: It is important to identify errors as early as possible and to communicate this identification to one's immediate superior. For the clinical chief, this is usually the vice president for medical affairs. In addressing the identified error, one should have the following concepts in place:

✦ A clear and precise description of the event and what led to the error.

✦ A determination of whether the error was one of commission or omission and what guidelines, procedures, or regulations, had they been applied, would have prevented the error.

✦ An assessment of the consequences of the error, including any relevant risk management issues.

✦ An assessment of the awareness of the error by the hospital community as well as the patients involved.

✦ An assessment of the perception of the error by the community and/or patients.

✦ A recommendation for correcting the damages.

✦ A recommendation for prevention of a future recurrence, including education, training, and/or evaluations.

✦ Any disciplinary action that may be warranted.

✦ A recommendation for public or internal statements with respect to the event.

Pitfall #10—Failing to buy into organizational values.

A manager who isn't philosophically and operationally committed to the mission and philosophy of the organization is going to be in generic conflict more often than not, or at least uncertain as to the reasons for what he or she is doing. One cannot be an effective manager or leader if one is in conflict with the organization's mission or objectives. This does not preclude disagreeing with decisions of institutional management. Nor does it preclude attempting to modify programs consistent with the mission or philosophy.

Failure to buy into the organizational value system will become apparent to the rest of the organization in a relatively short time, and the clinical chief will be labeled as such.

Strategy: The key to successful avoidance of this pitfall is acquiring a thorough knowledge of the mission statement and how it was derived. The clinical chief should assess his or her comfort level with the mission statement and the clinical philosophy of the institution. In the best of all possible worlds, the CEO and/or the vice president for medical affairs would have established with the clinical chief this comfort level before he or she committed to the job. Absent such an understanding, this should be one of the early strategic goals for the clinical chief. All challenges to programs or decisions should reflect an understanding and interpretation of the mission statement. Proposals and plans must convey the same approach.

Pitfall #11—Lack of availability.

Among the most common complaints about a supervisor in any organization is lack of availability. This refers not only to one's physical availability, but also one's receptivity to ideas, criticisms, and/or suggestions. It is also true that a manager may perceive him- or herself as available in contrast to the perception of his or her staff. If such perceptions persist, the staff will soon lose interest in trying to communicate with the manager, which ultimately leads to a loss of productivity and important feedback to the manager. Ultimately, this is destructive for both the manager and the staff. The timing, as well as the quality, of the response to staff input must be considered. Staff members tend to measure the availability of the manager by how promptly and with how much sensitivity a response is obtained.

Strategy: The first step is to establish clear guidelines to the members of one's staff as to how they are to reach you, whether it be in group meetings, one-to-one, by memoranda, or by verbal communication. The chief must indicate his or her style, that is, an open door or strictly by appointment. The style itself isn't as important as establishing a reputation for consistency and equal opportunity for staff. The more staff members perceive ease of access, the more readily they will communicate with the chief. Equally important is the perception that not only is it easy to make the communication, but also communications will be heard and respected. Prompt responses to queries will solidify the relationship between the chief and his or her staff. This is more important than whether the response is favorable or negative, because it allows the staff to move on with its responsibilities. It is equally important to be able to explain or justify negative responses, particularly in reference to the mission of the institution or specific adminis-trative strategies. Negative responses are more likely to be respected if the staff members have enough information to explain the response to their peers.

Pitfall #12—Failure to document performance.

One of the most important responsibilities of a manager is to monitor the performance of the staff. Communicating the findings of such monitoring to each individual staff member is the most effective way of sustaining and stimulating good performance. It also provides the mechanism for correcting and guiding an individual whose performance is deficient. To achieve these objectives, there must be accurate and consistent documentation of performance. One of the most difficult and stressful obligations of a clinical department chief is disciplinary action or criticism of a physician within the department. When such action is required, the absence of precise documentation and a record of reminders or warnings with respect to performance can nullify the objective of the chief's intervention. It also can result in risk to both the chief and the institution from a legal perspective.

Strategy: There should be a confidential file for every member of the department in which the chief keeps notes of both successes and problems. Acknowledging the achievements and successes of one's staff is easy to do but is often neglected. Indicating that such data are recorded is positive reinforcement to the staff. On the other hand, wherever problems are identified, it is even more critical that there be a clear documentation of date, time, place, witnesses, and whatever intervention was recommended. The record should contain notes or minutes of the discussions, be they a one-on-one criticism, a case review, a peer review, or a quality assurance finding. The goal should always be to educate the physician and change behavior, but if disciplinary action becomes necessary, it can only be effective with a well-documented record. Measures of performance should be as objective as possible. However, impressions and descriptive narrative are preferable to no information. Again, these data are part of the confidential file, but the chief may expect to have to review them with lawyers and/or risk managers when disputes over performance occur. When used for annual or periodic review of one's staff, these data can be shared individually.

Pitfall #13—Underestimating one's role in marketing the department and/or hospital.

There will be many measures of a clinical chief, such as successful patient care, scholarship, and contribution to the balance sheet of the hospital. Marketing the programs of one's department to the community has become a recognized responsibility of hospital managers. Hospital administrations and boards reasonably expect department chiefs to participate in this effort and to represent the hospital appropriately.

Strategy: In the course of "buying in" to the hospital's mission statement and the philosophy of the organization, the department chief can logically extend this commitment to the marketing effort. The successful clinical chief should acquire ease in marketing through his or her knowledge of the institution, its history, and its goals and objectives. The professional and material resources of the department, as well as its historical achievements, become the basis for promoting the department informally and formally within the medical and lay community. This should be coordinated with the strategies of the administration and the public relations department. Where the hospital has a formal marketing section, the theme for the marketing will be generated centrally. Otherwise, the initiative of the department for a marketing strategy should be presented to the vice president for medical affairs or the medical director, who can coordinate marketing efforts of all the clinical chiefs so that they are both complementary and consistent with an institutionwide effort.

Summation

This chapter has attempted to identify the typical pitfalls awaiting the new clinical department chief and to provide guidance for avoiding or overcoming them. The common theme that connects all of these exercises is the quality of communication, both vertically and horizontally, within the organization. Each potential conflict or road block has the potential for prevention. In each, prevention requires a clear understanding of organizational mission, relationships, expectations, and history. The position of clinical department chief is, for many physicians, a first step on the ladder of opportunities as a physician executive. One's growth and progress up that ladder requires being a student of organizational processes.

Robert A. Kramer, MD, is Executive Vice President, Newington Children's Hospital Foundation, Newington, Conn.

CHAPTER 8

Time Management

by Douglas P. Longenecker, MD

*T*here are as many experts in the field of time management as there are people who have written on the subject. In thinking of the management of time, it is perhaps more appropriate to consider personal management rather than time management. It is critical to balance personal versus professional time in any endeavor, whether medical practice, administrative medicine, or other professions.

Table 1, page 76, compares and contrasts practice time and administrative time for physicians. In the clinical arena, the physician's time is practice-driven. Time is consumed by the requirements of patients, procedures, paperwork, phone calls, mail, and third-party payers. Administratively, the physician's time is organizationally driven through meetings, interventions, plenary sessions, phone calls, mail, and administrative structure. Many other areas could be included in this list, but these are the most significant factors.

As can be determined by asking any patient waiting in a physician's office, physicians are perceived as poor time managers. Clinical practice dictates that time management be patient- and practice-driven. Consequently, a significant amount of activity falls in what may be described as the crisis arena. Even though many activities can, and must, be scheduled, because of the press on the physician's time from surgery, procedures, etc., a great deal of the practicing physician's time is driven by patients' needs and not by the physician. Physicians do not pay close attention to tight time allocations have gained the reputations of not only being late, but also being poor time managers.

There are specific differences between clinical and administrative time. In the clinical arena, as briefly listed above, time segments are largely patient- and schedule-driven, either by office visits or procedures. In the physician's administrative time, the system is management-driven. The administrative physician must be able to organize his or her time through self-discipline, have the time to interact with peer groups, and provide specific time for productive thinking and planning.

75

Table 1—Contrasts and Similarities of Practice vs. Administrative Time	
Clinical Practice (Patient Driven Needs)	**Administrative** (Organizationally Driven Needs)
1. Patients	1. Meetings
2. Procedures	2. Interventions
3. Paperwork	3. Plenary Sessions
4. Phone Calls	4. Phone Calls
5. Mail	5. Mail
6. Third Party Payers	6. Administrative Structure

To explore more closely the contrasts between clinical and administrative activity and time, let's look at an example of scheduling of clinical time.

Medical practice scheduling is well known to all physicians who have moved from a clinical to an administrative arena. Appropriate scheduling in a medical office or medical practice is dictated by the medical specialty. However, it is well known that the schedule may be constructed either in specific time blocks or on a wave method. Additionally, practice time is affected by specific procedures, be they surgical or other, related to outside scheduling availability. Appropriate staffing within the physician's office or practice arena is extremely important. Sufficient secretarial, nursing, and general office personnel are critical to an efficient medical practice. The layout of the office facility and of procedural rooms and the way the facility is equipped will greatly facilitate or hamper the physician's efficiency.

In administration, the physician must appropriate sufficient time for management. If the physician is both a practicing and an administrative physician, time must be rigorously scheduled for management activities. The support staff from an administrative aspect is equally important as the support staff from the physician's practice aspect. Because physicians in clinical practice commonly use their support staff for scheduling not only their office but also their procedural time, it is imperative for the administrative physician to effectively use his or her secretarial and administrative staff in an efficient manner.

Delegation of duties in both the clinical and the administrative arena is of utmost importance. This is accomplished through many mechanisms. However, the ability to specifically observe and supervise the delegation once it has happened is crucial. Administratively, this presents many problems for some physicians, as delegation to this depth is not frequently done in clinical practice.

In analyzing administrative and clinical physician's time, it is quite apparent that "something has to give." Management time can not be squeezed in between clinical activities. Management time must be specifically scheduled. It must be time that is used during a productive period of a physicians day. For most practicing physicians, the use of management time appears grossly inefficient when compared to clinical activities. As mentioned earlier, practicing physicians are familiar with the scheduling of patients and procedures for their clinical specialty. Most physician going from clinical practice to management positions are much less prepared for the scheduling of their time and allocation of priorities.

Table 2
Phases of Times Management
1. Notes/Check Lists
2. Calendars/Appointment Books
3. Prioritization of Time
4. Personal Management

A brief overview of the phases of time management are in order at this time (see table 2, left). The first phase may be described as developing notes and checklists to which frequent reference is made during the course of the day. The second phase would be the establishment of calendars and appointment books. The third phase is prioritization of time. This is apparent to all practicing physicians. A clinical example would be, given a busy office schedule, the time prioritization that would be required because of the appearance in the emergency department of a patient requiring immediate attention. Administrative time prioritization is somewhat different, but the basic elements are the same.

One must also recognize the fact that there are "crisis" interventions that are necessary throughout the course of an administrative day. This is frequently referred to as "putting out fires."

The fourth phase listed in table 2 is that of personal management. The concept of personal management changes one's philosophy from management of time to management of people. I can think of no better example of a paradigm shift than for a practicing physician to enter the administrative arena. Stephen Covey, in his book *The 7 Habits of Highly Effective People**, goes into great detail discussing paradigm shifts. He divides daily activities into four specific categories: urgent, nonurgent, important, and not important. He also describes, as shown by table 3, page 78, the interactions within the four quadrants. Quadrant I activities are crisis problems, pressing problems, and deadline-driven projects. Quadrant II activities are prevention, production capability activities, relationship building, recognizing new opportunities, planning, and recreation. Quadrant III activities are interruptions, some phone calls, mail, meetings, proximate pressing matters, and popular activities. Quadrant IV activities are trivia, busy work, some mail, some phone calls, time wasters, and pleasant activities. Quadrant IV activities are perceived by many managers to be wasted time.

---

* Covey, S. *The 7 Habits of Highly Effective People*. New York, N.Y.: Simon & Schuster, 1989.

Table 3

URGENT	NOT URGENT
IMPORTANT	
I **Activities:** Crises Pressing problems Deadline-driven projects	**II** **Activities:** Prevention, PC activities Relationship building Recognizing new opportunities Planning, recreation
NOT IMPORTANT	
III **Activities** Interruptions, some calls Some mail, some reports Some meetings Proximate, pressing matters Popular activities	**IV** **Activities** Trivia, busy work Some mail Some phone calls Time wasters Pleasant activities

To repeat, I can think of no better example of a paradigm shift than a practicing physicians assuming an administrative position. This is further exemplified by looking at table 3 in regard to clinical practice activities. Practicing physicians, on a daily basis, must deal with crises, pressing problems, and deadline-driven projects in their clinical activities. From an administrative aspect, Covey, and many others, feel it is extremely important to shift as many activities as possible into Quadrant II. This transition is a difficult task for the practicing physician. It requires the new administrative physician to change attitudes and philosophies, either totally or partially, from a clinical to an administrative posture (a paradigm shift). It has been shown that Quadrant I activities, to the exclusion of other activities, result in a high rate of stress, burnout, and crisis management. This is more graphically depicted in table 4, left.

Table 4

I Results:	II
• Stress • Burnout • Crisis management • Always putting out fires	IV
III	

In table 5, page 79, one can see that with physicians' predominant activity centered in Quadrant III activities, the results are short-term focus, crisis management activities, reputation of a chameleon character, and planning and goals of little value. The physician functioning in Quadrant III feels victimized, out of control, and shallow in relationships. Many clinical activities lie in Quadrant III, although they do not relate specifically to "out of control activities."

78

Table 5

I	II
III Results: • Short-term focus • Crisis management • Reputation-chameleon character • See goals and plans as worthless • Feel victimized, out of control • Shallow or broken relationships	**IV**

Table 6

I	II	
III	**IV Results:** • Total irresponsibility • Fired from job • Dependent on others • Dependent on others or institutions for basics	

Table 7

II	II
↑ ↑ ↑ ↑	← ← ← ← ← **Results:** • Vision, perspective • Balance • Discipline • Control • Few crises

Table 6, left, relates to Quadrant 4 activities, which can lead to total irresponsibility, termination from employment, total dependency on others, or dependency on institutions for basics. This behavior is contradictory to what a practicing physician must exhibit in his or her daily activities, as well as what he or she must produce in regard to administrative duties.

Activities located in Quadrant II—prevention, production capabilities, relationship building, recognizing new opportunities, planning, and even recreation—are the areas in which the administrative physician must focus his or her physical and intellectual energy. The results of these endeavors would be increase of vision and perspective, the balance of idealization, self-discipline, control, and diminution of administrative crises. These concepts are depicted in table 7, left.

Where the paradox occurs for the physician administrator relative to the clinical physician is the transferring of activities from Quadrant I to Quadrant II. It is a total impossibility for practicing physicians to transfer all of their activities to Quadrant II. In fact, it may be quite difficult for a predominance of clinical activities to be transferred to quadrant II because of the nature of clinical practice. Consequently, the physician who is engaged in both the clinical and the administrative fields of medicine must develop and maintain the ability to "shift gears" or "paradigms" between the administrative Quadrant II and the clinical quadrant I activities.

This concept may be expressed by contrasting proactivity versus reactivity. The clinical physician, by the nature of the profession of medicine, must be a reactive individual. The clinical physician must be able to deal with crisis/pressing problems, to shift his or her thinking immediately to the problems at hand, and to plan for the long-term aspect of clinical care.

For the administrative physician, conversely, it is much more appropriate and effective if the proactive mode is employed to produce decisions.

To use a more specific example of the reactive versus proactive mode, the practicing physician needs to see patients either at his or her office or at the hospital. The physician must immediately form the most appropriate plan of action and envision medical needs to arrive at a correct judgment. In contrast, the administrative physician faced with a decision should become proactive rather than reactive, because there may be more than one decision that would be appropriate. Furthermore, in an administrative situation, the physician must look at alternatives to a much greater extent, especially in regard to the people that surround and work with him or her in the administrative environment.

In summary, in time management or, more specifically, in personal management, it is apparent that clinical thought processes and administrative decisions may diverge in concept. In addition to the divergence of clinical and administrative physician activity, one must look at the support staff of the practicing physician as well as the of administrative physician. Practicing physicians are accustomed to delegating less critical responsibilities in both the office and the hospital setting. Practicing physicians ask their office nursing personnel, their front office employees, and hospital-based technicians and nurses to assist them in their activities by the delegation of appropriate responsibilities. There is a deeper level of responsibility to be delegated from an administrative position. The administrator must have well-trained and capable individuals who are in a position not only to carry out decisions by the administrator, but also to formulate ideas, concepts, and decision making processes on their own.

For some physicians, it is difficult to accept the delegation of this level of responsibility, but this is a mandated conceptual change or "paradigm shift" for the administrative physician. Practicing physician have no choice but to reserve significant clinical decisions for themselves, to the exclusion of delegation. In contrast, it is the ineffective physician manager who feels that he or she is the only individual who can make decisions or perform the procedures necessary for an appropriate administrative functioning.

These concepts are important for the full-time physician administrator, but perhaps more significant for the part-time physician administrator. The changes in thought processes and conceptual insights from a clinical "action" mode to an administrative "delegating" mode are difficult transitions to make.

It is important for the physician administrator, particularly physicians just leaving clinical practice to join administration, to be understand and accept that:

✦ Time interactions and time utilization present difficulties.

✦ Administrative physicians cannot expect the immediate gratification seen in clinical practice and must be able to expect and accept long-term gratification.

✦ Individual decisions are not final, as they are in clinical practice.

✦ Organizational structure and actions are the basis for administrative medicine.

Douglas P. Longenecker, MD, is Vice President, Medical Affairs, Good Samaritan Hospital and Health Center, Dayton, Ohio.

CHAPTER 9

The Economics and Fiscal Management of Provider Organizations

by Hugh W. Long, PhD, JD, and James D. Suver, DBA, CMA

Introduction

Fiscal or financial management covers a broad spectrum of activities associated with the economics of an organization. Fiscal management encompasses everything from recording (writing down) in monetary terms actual historical organizational activity, to determining any one of a number of possible "costs" of a product or unit of service, to raising money for short-term or long-term purposes, to forecasting an unknown future economic environment for the purpose of allocating scarce resources today among competing alternative uses.

The purposes of this chapter are:

✦ To introduce you to some very basic aspects of fiscal management and what various fiscal specialists do.

✦ To provide you some familiarity with internal fiscal information, financial statements, and the uses of each.

✦ To give you some understanding of the economics that underlie organizational financing and resource allocation decisions.

Fiscal Management—Types, Roles, Functions

The two major branches of fiscal management within organizations are *accounting* and *finance*. "To account" means "to keep a record of," but, although that is a big part of accounting activity, accounting encompasses a great deal more than simply keeping records. "To finance" means to bring together monetary resources for some particular purpose (meet a payroll, buy a piece of equipment), but finance involves a great deal more than simply bringing together piles of money.

Accounting and finance are very different from each other. Each of these fiscal areas has distinct uses and applications, and each is built on a quite separate and different collection of concepts and assumptions. As discussed below, using finance cash-flow concepts to define "income" would be as misleading as using financial accounting mechanisms for asset acquisition decisions. Serious errors, indeed irrational outcomes, would result. Hence, identifying the distinct characteristics and uses of each area is a major priority for managers.

Accounting and Accounting Systems

The field of accounting involves many subspecialties. Internal to health care (and other business) organizations, one finds *financial accounting* and *managerial* and/or *cost accounting*. Financial accounting has the primary role of keeping records and preparing financial statements; managerial accounting addresses budgeting and control issues; and cost accounting identifies costs throughout the organization, distributing (allocating) those costs to various services or programs (units of output). Other accounting subspecialties include actuaries, who make statistical predictions about the frequency with which certain events (e.g., number of births during a one-year period for a specified population group) may take place; tax accountants, who specialize in working with the income tax code and regulations; and, in the health care industry, accountants who specialize in the technical aspects of health insurance and payment systems. Accounting firms use certified public accountants (CPAs) to audit the financial statements of client organizations to certify the validity of those statements in accordance with certain rules. CPAs, and often certified management accountants (CMAs), also provide consulting services related to the fiscal management of the organization.

Every day, a typical health care organization (1) writes checks to suppliers (e.g., employees, utility companies, independent contractors, vendors) of the resources consumed in delivering past, current, or future patient services; (2) delivers patient services, and (3) receives and deposits payments for future, current, or past patient services. The accounting system collects information about all of these transactions (and, indeed, itself is responsible for some of them). As the repository of such information, the accounting system is obviously the institutional component that can collate and organize this information for both external and internal decision makers.

Managers must have timely and accurate data about organizational revenue, collections, expenses, costs, and asset values in order to exercise proper fiscal control over the provider entity. External parties (e.g., lenders, owners, payers) also need prompt and accurate information about organizational performance. The accounting system is the primary method for accomplishing these objectives. Basically, an accounting system consists of methods and procedures for collecting, segregating, and summarizing individual transactions that occur during a specified period.

Accounting information must be reported in sufficient detail to allow decision makers to make appropriate judgments about the various dimensions of organizational performance—for example, are revenues covering expenses?

Also important is the timeliness of information. Detailed, comprehensive financial reports are not of much use if they are presented too late to be included in the decision-making process. For example, monthly expense reports that are presented three to four weeks after the close of the operating period are of little help to managers in controlling the current month's expenses. And lenders will be disinclined to advance monies to an organization for which the most recent financial statements are eight months old.

As is the case with most real world activities, the design and operation of accounting systems involve trade-offs. Organizations must balance detail and accuracy on the one hand, and timeliness on the other, keeping an eye on the costs of each.[1]

Figure 1, below, shows rule-of-thumb reporting time frames for a sampling of internal and external reports. The availability of computer-assisted data collection makes it feasible to provide more timely and lower cost financial statements and statistical records than under earlier manual systems.[2]

Figure 1. Sample Reporting Times*

Volume of Services	Daily	Due on daily basis by payer classification
Cash Flow	Weekly	Due every Tuesday
Full-time Employees	Biweekly	Due following working day after each budgeted personnel payroll period
Budget Comparison	Monthly	Due tenth working day after end of month
Variance Analysis	Monthly	Due tenth working day after end of month
Interim Income Statement	Quarterly	Due tenth working day after end of quarter
Balance Sheet	Annual	NLT 60 days after end of fiscal year
Statements of "Cash Flow"	Annual	NLT 60 days after end of fiscal year
Income Statement	Annual	NLT 60 days after end of fiscal year

* Other schedules can be used to report on key areas. For example:
- Aging of Accounts Receivable
- Inventory levels
- Patient origin by Zip Code
- Sources of in-referrals/admissions

---

[1] As an example of striving to achieve such a balance affecting internal controls, management might choose to monitor only certain key areas—levels of service volume, payer mix, salary expenses, supply levels and expenses—and receive more timely reports on just these areas. Each manager should develop key indicators and receive reports accordingly.

[2] Computerization also makes it feasible to collect accounting information from a number of perspectives simultaneously, e.g., from the point of view of responsibility centers, "product" lines, services, procedures, etc., in sufficient detail to enrich greatly the quality of managerial decision making.

Financial Accounting.

The financial accountant is charged with recording actual and fiscal activities of the organization. In effect, financial accounting writes a fiscal history of the organization according to a particular set of rules.[3] That history records everything that happens in the organization that is measurable in dollars. The keeping of that history book involves bookkeeping, the mechanical side of financial accounting. Bookkeeping includes the maintenance of paper or electronic journals and ledgers, the entries to which are called *debits* and *credits*.[4]

In order to keep books that present a consistent and reasonable picture of the past, financial accounting attempts to associate dollar values with real physical events as nearly in time to the occurrence of those events as possible. To facilitate this, accountants use the concept of an *accrual*, one of the most basic accounting notions. Accrual accounting is the process by which dollar values are assigned to activities in a way that links those values to the output (services) of the organization and to the timing of the organization's production of those services.

For example, in accrual accounting, *revenue* is a concept used to describe the value of services delivered to a patient, not the receipt of cash associated with that delivery. Accountants *recognize* revenue when the service is delivered. For example, in a fee-for-service setting (or in a prepaid setting when services are provided to someone who is not a member of the prepaid plan), a physician who sees a patient confirms the services delivered by entering information (e.g., a CPT code) on a piece of paper or in a computer. This information is received by the accounting function to begin the process of billing the patient for a deductible, for a copayment, or for the rendering of a product or service not otherwise covered by prepayment or insurance, and the process of triggering payments from third parties. As soon as that happens, the accountant *recognizes* the associated revenue. The patient visit has occurred, the encounter has taken place, service has been rendered, revenue is recognized. It is not critical to the accounting process whether or not the provider organization has *collected* for the service. As long as it is reasonable to expect that payment will be received, it does not matter when those dollars come in the door. The service has taken place, and, if you want to keep a record of that, you recognize the revenue associated with service immediately. The same accrual concept applies to expenses associated with that service. The cost of the resources directly attributable to producing that service will be recognized at the time service is delivered. That cost (or expense) may include resources used, even though payment for those resources has not yet been made. It may also include resources that have already been paid for. Regardless of the timing of payment for such resources, however, the accountant will recognize the cost of the resources used in delivering the service during and only during the period services are actually delivered.

---

[3] Most organizations follow guidelines and procedures established by the Financial Accounting Standards Board (FASB) or Government Accounting Standards Board (GASB), the Securities Exchange Commissions (SEC), and the American Institute of Certified Public Accountants (AICPA).

[4] Debits are entries on left-hand side of the ledger logs and credits are entries on the right-hand side.

One especially important example of this shifting through time of cost attribution is the case of recognizing historical outlays by a mechanism the accountant calls "depreciation."[5] If the organization acquires a $100,000 piece of equipment and expects it to last five years, delivering service throughout that period, and having no salvage value at the end of the five years, and if applicable reporting rules call for using "straight-line" depreciation, the accountant will charge off that $100,000 expenditure by recording a $20,000 expense each year for the next five years. The intent is to allocate the cost of the equipment to the several intervals of time within its entire useful life. This concept of accounting depreciation spreads the cost of capital (real) assets over their useful lives, time-coincident with use for the delivery of service. If the organization has interest expense (as it would if it had borrowed money to make the equipment purchase), that interest expense will be recognized as an expense in the period when it is due, because the interest is attributable to the use of the borrowed money over the life of the debt.

A further characteristic of the financial accounting process is that it presumes that "all dollars are created equal." That is, accounting treats $100 of revenue in January exactly the same as it treats $100 of revenue in December. This ignores (intentionally) differential purchasing power of dollars at various times and "opportunity costs" (the fact that funds received earlier can be invested or used in other ways). The reason accounting does this is largely historical. While there are more economically correct ways of writing down historical numbers, they are intrinsically complex. The accrual accounting approach has the advantage of being a less complex and standardized way of recording transactions that is quite adequate for many purposes.

Certain formal amalgamations of recorded transactions are known as Income Statements, Balance Sheets, and Statements of "Cash Flow." A discussion of these standard financial statements and their interpretation appears in Appendix A to this chapter. These statements are designed to present an internally consistent picture of historical organizational activity in accordance with a very specifically defined point of view, a set of rules known as "Generally Accepted Accounting Principles" (GAAP).

GAAP is generated by the accounting profession through its Financial Accounting Standards Board (FASB). FASB, in concert with the SEC in certain matters, decrees that GAAP is the rules of the game for writing the fiscal history book.[6] The rules specify, within limits, how you record prepaid insurance, how you treat salvage value, how you depreciate or amortize an asset, etc. The rules tell you that how you record interest during construction of buildings is different from how you treat interest during ongoing delivery of services. GAAP tells you how to account for mergers, acquisitions, subsidiaries, holding companies,

---

[5] If the outlay was for certain types of physical assets, we use the term "depreciation:" for certain intangible assets, the term we use is "amortization."

[6] For public sector entities, a parallel set of rules is the responsibility of GASB, the Government Accounting Standards Board.

something called "goodwill," and almost any other complication you can think of. GAAP is a technical set of rules designed to allow financial accountants to present a consistent, uniform fiscal picture via formal financial statements.

The importance of these concepts is not in the specifics of GAAP but rather in the fact that *a formal, written set of rules exists that accountants must apply*. These rules are, in effect, the *standards of practice* for accountants. And, in general, the "better" the accountant, the more seriously he or she will take these standards. Serious application of these standards maintains the integrity and the comparability (both through time and across organizations) of "the books."

There are, of course, many judgment calls made by the CPA in the application of GAAP, for there are always gray areas. This is one of the reasons we have external audits. Outside CPAs, guided in audit procedures by standards established by the American Institute of Certified Public Accountants (AICPA), check the work of an organization's financial accountants and formally attest to adherence (or lack thereof) to GAAP in the presentation of the organization's financial statements. Fundamentally, this system allows you to rely on financial statements constructed in accordance with GAAP and attested to by a CPA auditor and in order to determine some very important things. The attest statement by the external CPA provides assurance to the reader of the financial statements that GAAP has been followed consistently from year to year in the reporting of financial information.

For a single organization, looking at its audited financial statements through time allows you (without knowing anything else about the organization) to draw reasonably strong conclusions about that organization's fiscal status, because you can rely on the statements following the rules of the game. Also, you can take sets of financial statements from similar organizations, all for the same period, put them side by side, and make relatively strong comparative statements about the relative fiscal positions of those organizations.

Thus, while all financial statements produced by the financial accounting system are important to internal users, audited financial statements are very important to "external" users, such as boards of directors, bankers, or numerous government entities. A few tools that are useful in analyzing financial statements are also presented in Appendix A to this chapter.

Managerial and Cost Accounting.
As important as the statements produced by financial accounting systems are, other analyses of the information amassed by the accounting system are even more important for internal managerial purposes. In addition, organizations typically engage in various extensions of financial accounting activity in the form of cost accounting and budgeting. Although cost accounting is sometimes viewed as a subset of managerial accounting, managerial and cost accounting together deal with formulating budgets, analyzing actual fiscal performance in comparison to what was budgeted, projecting the effects of management deci-

sions on future financial accounting statements, identifying actual costs of producing services, calculating "full" costs of services using cost allocation formulas, and dealing with other related issues of cost and payment (e.g., internal transfer pricing, income distribution mechanisms, maximizing third-party payments related to cost). The sections that follow offer a survey of managerial and cost accounting activities.

Budgeting

✦ The Budgeting Process

The budgeting process and the resulting output, the approved master budget, are probably among the most valuable short-term tools available to the manager. An effective master budget defines the plan of action that management has approved for the next year of operation. It expresses the goals and objectives of the organization in quantitative terms. The master budget consists of the following components:

— The operating budget, composed of revenue and expense categories.

— The capital budget, comprising investment decisions on long-term assets, such as equipment and facilities.

— The cash budget, which traces the inflow and outflow of cash resources and identifies when borrowing is needed and when excess cash is available for investments.

— Pro forma financial statements, which represent what the financial condition of the institution will be at the end of the budget year if the plan is followed.

The components of the master budget cycle are illustrated in Figure 2, page 90. A discussion of basic budgeting techniques appears in Appendix B to this chapter.

✦ Benefits

Preparation of the budget and the resulting approved document can result in the following benefits to the organization:

— Communication is improved throughout the organization. If the budget reflects the goals and objectives of the organization, the preparers and readers of the document will know these objectives. Through its allocation of resources, the budget communicates what is important.

— Coordination is improved, because the completed master budget ensures that all preparers are working with the same data on anticipated patient loads and expenses. Estimated demand and services to be supplied are made explicit.

— Control is improved, because the budget authorizes certain levels of expenses and clarifies what revenues are to be anticipated. Comparison with actual results enables management to become aware of deviations from the budget as they occur.

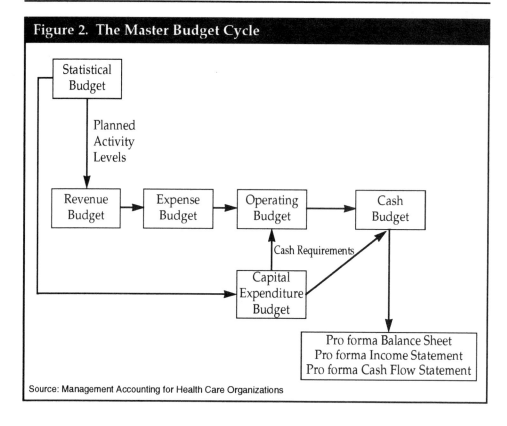

Figure 2. The Master Budget Cycle

Source: Management Accounting for Health Care Organizations

— Motivation is improved, because people who have participated in the budget feel a greater loyalty to the organization. They know what is anticipated and what is expected of them.

—Finally, comparison of the plan with actual results facilitates performance management. Variances can be computed to focus management interest on results not in accordance with the budget.

✦ **Requirements**
To achieve the benefits listed above, certain activities must be accomplished:

— Top management of the facility must be involved with and committed to the budgeting process. The completed plan must be used for decision-making.

— There should be a formal system with well-defined goals and objectives, formalized reports, and responsibility accounting. Training sessions for supervisors and department heads are usually necessary to provide the proper guidance and motivation.

— Sufficient time should be allowed for preparation, negotiation, and review by interested parties. Typically, a minimum of 90 days should be scheduled for the budget process.

— Supervisors with responsibility for cost control and/or revenue generation should be actively involved in preparation of the budget. This joint effort ensures that the budget is a participating budget, not just a management budget.

— Finally, there should be accurate data for expense and revenue projections and a statistical base in terms of work and dollars involved. For example, reimbursement levels from third-party payers must be anticipated and used in the budget plan. Formal recognition of these constraints will make the budget more realistic and useful for planning purposes. The inflation rate must be estimated and included in the planned expenses for the next period. Inflation rates should be determined for each major cost element, such as salaries, food, utilities, supplies, etc., in order to obtain the best possible expense budget.

✦ Budgetary Control

Budgets cannot control costs; only people can control costs. The budget, by itself, is only a tool to help managers and supervisors make decisions. An effective process will involve all levels of management and supervision in the preparation of the budget. However, because of the dynamic nature of providing health care services, performance information must also be provided periodically to those same managers and supervisors if corrective action is to be taken. Timely budget reporting provides this information.

An effective budget reporting system provides information using a responsibility center concept. For example, the budget report received by a manager or supervisor would identify those costs that are controllable by that individual. For revenue centers, the report would focus on the contribution margin or the difference between revenues and expenses. The purpose is to encourage provision of services in ways that will enhance the total dollar amount of the contribution margin.

✦ Summary

Reports must be designed to meet the needs of the user. What is appropriate for one organization may not be effective for another. The level of detail, the type of information, and the timeliness of the report depend on the management training and the style of the manager.

Cost Concepts
✦ Cost Behavior

Preparation of a budget requires a basic understanding of cost behavior in relation to volume and, as will be discussed later, in terms of responsibility centers. Costs can be expressed as they relate to changes in activities, such as occupancy rates, patient visits, patient mix, services provided, etc. Costs described in terms of activity levels (volume) are usually separated in terms of fixed and variable components. A fixed cost is a cost that does not change

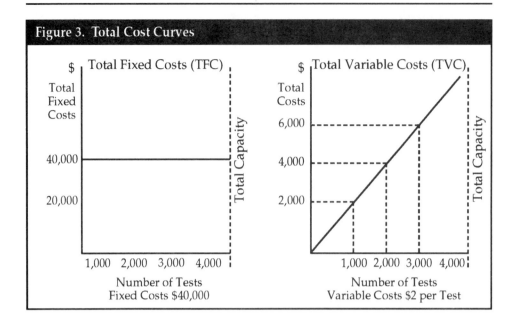

Figure 3. Total Cost Curves

Total Fixed Costs (TFC)
Fixed Costs $40,000

Total Variable Costs (TVC)
Variable Costs $2 per Test

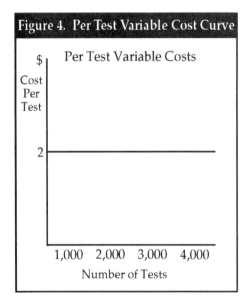

Figure 4. Per Test Variable Cost Curve

Per Test Variable Costs

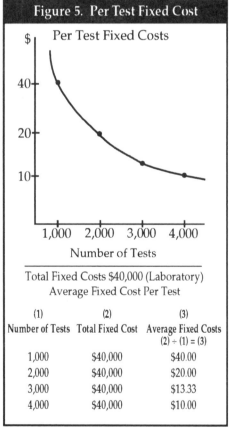

Figure 5. Per Test Fixed Cost

Per Test Fixed Costs

Total Fixed Costs $40,000 (Laboratory)
Average Fixed Cost Per Test

(1) Number of Tests	(2) Total Fixed Cost	(3) Average Fixed Costs (2) ÷ (1) = (3)
1,000	$40,000	$40.00
2,000	$40,000	$20.00
3,000	$40,000	$13.33
4,000	$40,000	$10.00

92

within the relevant range of alternative levels of activity.[7] For example, the manager's salary will not typically change with the number of patients. This does not mean it cannot be changed, but it changes as a function of management decisions rather than of activity level. Variable costs, on the other hand, are costs that vary directly with volume. For example, raw food costs will vary with the number of meals served; the costs of drugs and pharmacy items can vary with the number of procedures performed; etc. These types of costs are illustrated graphically in Figure 3, page 92.

The manager must work with per unit comparisons in addition to the total cost approach displayed in Figure 3. Costs are typically expressed on a per unit basis for reimbursement, rate setting, and billing activities. Just as we view total costs as the combination of variable and fixed costs, total costs per unit are a combination of variable costs per unit and fixed costs per unit. On a per unit basis, variable costs are the same for each individual unit of service. For example, if the variable costs for one test are $2.00, they are $4.00 for two tests, $6.00 for three tests, etc. Of course, the average or per unit cost remains at $2.00 regardless of volume. This cost relationship can be expressed graphically, as shown in Figure 4, page 92.

In determining the total per unit cost, the determination of the fixed cost component presents a more difficult challenge, complicated by the large proportion that fixed costs represent of total costs in the health care industry. Because fixed costs per unit are obtained by dividing total fixed costs by the level of activity, the more units provided, the lower the fixed costs per unit. Continuing our test example above, suppose the laboratory supervisor is paid $40,000. At a volume of 1,000 tests, this calculates to $40 per test. But the fixed costs per unit for 2,000 tests would be $40,000 divided by 2,000, or $20 per test. As most experienced managers have observed, the volume of tests is of vital concern for financial well-being because of the heavy fixed cost nature of most health care services. The relationship of per unit fixed costs to volume is illustrated in Figure 5, page 92.

✦ Average (Full) Cost Determination
The determination of what a test costs is typically based on the average cost of providing the test (Total Cost divided by Volume = Average Cost, where Total Cost = Total Variable Costs + Total Fixed Costs]. As discussed above, fixed costs per unit will vary as the level of output or volume changes. Therefore, it is impossible to determine per unit costs without first estimating the level of output. For example, Figure 6, page 94, presents an analysis of the laboratory example discussed above in which capacity is now assumed to be 8,000 tests for the period of time covered by the analysis.

---

[7] The relevant range of activity is typically the maximum capacity of the organization, using existing resources to deliver the service being analyzed within the period of time covered by the analysis. Should the provider decide to meet demand in excess of that capacity, additional capacity costs would have to be incurred. (Such additonal costs themselves, would almost always be fixed over the additional range of volume those costs would create.) In other words, no fixed cost is absolutely fixed.

Figure 6. Average (Full) Cost Determination

(1) Estimated Number of Tests	(2) Average Variable Cost	(3) Average Fixed Cost $40,000 ÷ Col. (1)	(4) Full Cost Per Test Col. (2) + Col. (3)
1,000	$2	$40.00	$42.00
2,000	2	$20.00	$22.00
3,000	2	$13.33	$15.33
4,000	2	$10.00	$12.00
5,000	2	$ 8.00	$10.00
6,000	2	$ 6.67	$ 8.67
7,000	2	$5.71	$7.71
8,000	2	$5.00	$7.00

Figure 7. Responsibility Center Reporting

Department Activities for the Month of May 199x

	Dollars	Percentage
Net Revenues	$ 3,000	100
Controllable Operating Expenses		
Variable Costs	450	15
Contribution Margin	$ 2,550	85
Controllable Fixed Costs	$ 2,280	76
Controllable Operating Margin	$ 270	9
Allocated Costs	1,500	50
Net Operating Margin (Loss)	**($ 1,230)**	**(41)**

Figure 8. Sample Report of Test Activity Measures

Capacity	Budget	Actual	Variance	Budget as % of Capacity	Actual as % of Capacity
110	100	90	10	91%	82%

Computation of full costs per unit is an important element in establishing prices or rates. That computation depends on the planned fixed cost and estimated volume, because the variable cost component is usually not sensitive to changes in the level of output within the relevant range of output. Hence, if one wants to establish a price or rate that covers the costs (in total or per test), that price or rate necessarily embodies/relies upon the underlying fixed cost and volume assumptions.

✦ Related Cost Definitions

Management must be aware of cost classifications in addition to the fixed and variable cost behavior dichotomy. One of the more useful categorizations is direct and indirect costs. Direct costs can be traced directly to the cost objective being measured. For example, the variable cost of the lab test and the cost of the supervisor are both direct costs of the tests. Conversely, costs that are necessary but are not directly involved with the test are indirect costs. Examples of indirect costs include senior management salaries and the cost of running the business office. These are part of the total cost of providing the test, but, because they cannot be traced directly to the test (and, in fact, support other outputs in addition to this test), they must be *allocated* to this test through some mechanism. The distinction between direct and indirect costs is crucial in responsibility accounting and reporting. By separating costs into direct and indirect categories, managers and supervisors can be held accountable for those costs they can control. An example of this type of report is illustrated in Figure 7, page 94.

In Figure 7, even though an overall loss is reported, we can see that in terms of direct costs over which departmental personnel have control, a $270 positive controllable operating margin has been achieved.

It is also important to have timely reports on the differences between planned and actual volume of services provided. Because of the interaction between volume and fixed costs in determining per unit costs, it is important for management to know how the volume of services actually provided differs from the budgeted volume. This type of report is shown in Figure 8, page 94, and can be expressed in units or in percentage of budgeted amount.

Analysis of incremental costs is particularly useful for management decision making. The incremental cost concept is that the only costs relevant to a decision are those that change as a result of the decision. For example, in deciding between two blood analyzers for the laboratory, the cost of the supervisor of blood work would not be a factor unless it varied between the two alternatives. Similarly, the salary of the laboratory director and other indirect administrative costs would not be included in the analysis.

Another important cost concept is the opportunity cost. Basically, opportunity costs are the benefits that would be realized if alternatives to the course of action being recommended were adopted. For example, opportunity costs exist when Test A is done instead of Test B. Opportunity costs are the revenues net of expenses forgone by not doing Test B.

Another cost category, sunk costs, reflects decisions that have already been made and cannot be changed by new decisions. Typical sunk costs are past expenditures for equipment: costs that have been capitalized. Capitalized costs represent assets that cannot be written off in the year of purchase according to generally accepted accounting principles. Typically, they are assets that are expected to produce benefits in more than one operating period. They are converted to expenses by means of periodic depreciation charges. Over the useful life of the assets, depreciation charges result in the recognition of the purchase price of the asset as a noncash expense against the revenue of the facility. The amount of the asset that is undepreciated is shown on the balance sheet as a net asset, the historical cost minus the accumulated depreciation charges. This net amount is called the book value of the asset.

The replacement of old equipment with new equipment would typically result in the removal/liquidation of the old equipment. If the old equipment still had an undepreciated book value of $2,000, this $2,000 should not be considered in a purchase decision. The $2,000 cost will be the same under any alternative, replacement or not, and the $2,000 book value will be written off either as a depreciation expense (if not replaced) or, in most cases, as a capital loss (if it is replaced). In either case, the $2,000 cost remains the same. If the timing of the write off affects taxes or third-party payment, that second-order effect would be incremental to the decision and should be considered because of time value of money considerations discussed in the finance section later in this chapter.

✦ **Cost Estimating Techniques**
Considerable progress has been made in the recent past in applying statistical modeling to estimate costs and cost behavior in for health care settings. Most of these techniques involve a form of regression analysis in which independent variables such as patient days are used to predict dependent variables such as nursing hours and supply costs on the basis of historical relationships. For example, a relationship between volume of laboratory tests and supervisory hours could be presented on a scatter diagram as shown in Figure 9, page 98. The relatively flat nature of the curve indicates that supervisory hours are fixed for the range of tests covered. The slope of the regression line in Figure 10, page 98, indicates that technician hours do increase with tests, as common sense would suggest. Supervisors are involved with administration and supervision of the technicians, while the technicians perform most of the direct work. Statistical techniques can be used to estimate the fixed and variable portion of the technician hours.

Managers who wish to explore these techniques in greater detail are encouraged to review the references for this section at the end of this chapter.

✦ **Overhead Costs**
Overhead or indirect costs can represent a significant part of the total costs of the health care provider. Costs that cannot be traced directly to the provision of individual patient services typically fall into the overhead area. The salaries of senior management, clerical staff, accounting staff, general maintenance/housekeeping costs are examples of overhead costs. These costs are difficult to control, because, while they are necessary, they are typically not directly related to the provision of a patient service. Thus, they do not directly provide revenues to the institution.

In addition, because there is no direct relationship between revenues and costs, it is difficult to determine what should be the "correct" amount of these costs, i.e., when should they be expanded or when should they be cut? What *should* be the size of a business office? How many accountants, clerks, administrators are needed? What type of equipment do they require? How much space should be allotted to them?

These decisions—and their resultant costs—are not directly related to the number of patient visits, the number of discharges, or the number of procedures performed, but they are an essential part of providing high-quality service to patients. In order to determine the full cost of providing services, it is necessary to devise some method of allocating a "fair" share of the overhead costs to each activity being performed.

✦ Allocation Methods

Allocation of overhead costs to the various activities of the organization requires development of an overhead charge per unit of service. Overhead charges are basically "average" shares of total overhead costs that can be applied to the service performed. Total overhead costs can be determined from the budget before the period of operation begins and from the accounting system after the period of operation ends. These total overhead costs are divided by the activity base selected to obtain the overhead charge (total overhead costs divided by volume). Each unit of service receives an estimated share of the overhead cost through this average rate. For example, business office costs could be allocated on the basis of the number of employees in each section. Nursing administration costs could be allocated according to the number of FTE nurses or the level of patient activity. Social service costs could be allocated according to the number of users or the total hours of service received by each patient.

Allocation of overhead requires that the health care provider be divided into patient care centers and patient support centers. Patient care centers are the departments that provide direct care and for which revenue can be recognized. Support centers are all other activities or cost centers, such as the business office, housekeeping, or marketing.

✦ Summary

In order to determine what a service or an activity costs, it is necessary to define exactly the purpose for which the cost information is being collected. Because of the effect of fixed costs on per unit costs, such cost figures are appropriate only for the volume selected. Statistical techniques are available to assist managers in estimating costs and cost behavior. Overhead costs present special challenges, and choices surrounding overhead allocations can significantly affect calculated per unit total costs.

Figure 9. Relative Value Units and Rate Determination

Test/ Procedure	(1) RVUs Procedure	(2) Budgeted Procedures	(3) Total Budgeted RVUs	(4) Revenue* Indicators	(5) Charge per Procedure	Total Revenue per Procedure
			(1) x (2)		(1) x (4)	(2) x (5)
A	2	200	400	$8.50	$17.00	$3,400
B	3	500	1,500	8.50	25.50	12,750
C	1	1,000	1,000	8.50	8.50	8,500
D	5	400	2,000	8.50	42.50	17,000
E	3	2,000	6,000	8.50	25.50	51,000
F	1	900	900	8.50	8.50	7,650
		5,000	11,800			$100,300

*Department Financial Requirements $100,300
(Total Department Revenue Needed)

Divided by Total Budgeted
Department RVUs (Units of Service)   11,800

Equals Revenue Indicator $8.50

Figure 10.

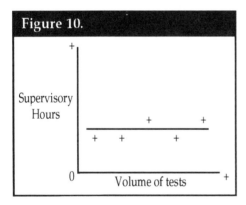

Supervisory Hours

Volume of tests

Figure 11.

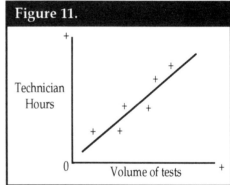

Technician Hours

Volume of tests

Standard Costs

Standard costs represent what a service or procedure should cost given realistic efficiency goals and current cost information. For example, if RN costs are expected to be $12 an hour next year and the patient mix is expected to require 3.5 RN hours per patient day, the standard RN cost per patient day would be $42.00. Deviations from this amount would need to be explained. Similar standards could be developed for dietary, laundry, housekeeping, maintenance, and supplies. Standard costs are preplanned and can be a natural output of the budgeting process. By carefully computing standard costs, benchmarks can be established for monitoring expenditures over the course of the operating year. The difference between actual costs and standard costs is called a variance. A variance could be caused by a change either in the cost of the items purchased or in the amount used. An analysis of variances can be an effective management tool in controlling expenses and rewarding responsible supervisors. Appendix C to this chapter provides a more detailed discussion of standard costing techniques and variance analysis.

Rate Setting Techniques

Health care organizations provide a variety of services to their patients. In some cases, the rate or the payment for the service is determined by third-party payers. On other occasions, the charge is determined by competition. In most cases, as a matter of policy, management and the board of trustees or directors will decide what rate should be established. Typically, these rates are based on full costs (defined in the preceding section as the variable costs of providing the service, direct fixed costs, and a fair share of the overhead or higher level fixed costs) and the desired (profit) margin. This average charge could be determined by dividing the total cost of providing the service plus desired profit by the estimated volume of service to be provided. From the above relationships, the importance of the volume factor should be evident. The greater the volume of services provided, the lower the charge can be. A more thorough discussion of cost/volume/profit relationships appears in Appendix D to this chapter.

Another approach to rate setting uses intensity-based information. For example, in departments such as radiology or occupational therapy, where relative value units or other intensity-of-care indicators are available, it is possible to develop the rates to be charged if the number of procedures by type of intensity are known. Figure 11, page 98, illustrates a department where several different types of procedures must be performed. The appropriate charge and the planned budget are developed on the basis of the mix of procedures and total financial requirements.

Finance

Finance focuses on matters quite different from those addressed by accounting. Accounting primarily deals with reporting an organization's historical activity in fiscal terms and secondarily makes forecasts of future financial statements and performance. Finance, in contrast to accounting, is exclusively future-oriented and deals with fiscal decision-making as to sources of financing and resource allocation (uses of financing). Both accounting and financial make important contributions to managerial processes, but they are also very different from each other.

For example, while accounting tries to match dollar figures with *physical* events, such as "patients served," finance matches dollar figures only with *fiscal* events, such as the collection of monies for services to patients. As a result, finance is concerned with the accounting accrual concept in only peripheral ways. Finance focuses not on when the service delivery occurs but, rather, on when money associated with that service comes in or goes out the door. Are you going to collect tomorrow, next week, or two months from now? Are you ever going to collect?

When does the *cash flow* occur? Similarly, finance does not associate resource cost with the timing of resource use, but rather with the timing of the payment for the resource. Finance focuses on receipts, not revenue, and on expenditures, not expenses or costs. This is because it is concerned with *future* cash flows or their equivalents, not past performance.

Suppose that you order a diagnostic laboratory test today that is performed today and a corresponding charge is generated at the same time. Assume further that medical supplies already on hand were used to obtain and to test the specimen. The accountant will recognize the revenues from the test today, whether or not any collection occurred today. If there was no collection, the accountant will recognize a corresponding increase in "accounts receivable" on the balance sheet. Finance will recognize nothing until the actual collection occurs. The accountant will recognize the "expense" of the supplies today, reducing an "inventory" (of supplies) account on the balance sheet. Finance will recognize nothing today unless there is a cash outlay today for those supplies.[8] Finance is interested in and will recognize only actual cash inflows and outflows, regardless of when the economic activity that gives rise to those flows takes place.

Finance also treats capital expenditures very differently from the way they are treated by accounting. If you decide to spend $100,000 for a piece of equipment that is expected to be productively employed for five years, the $100,000 is gone as soon as you acquire the equipment. Finance "recognizes" the full "cost" of the equipment when the cash outflow for the equipment takes place. It does not matter if the machine is going to last two years, five years, or 10 years. What the accountant will write down under the label "depreciation" in years hence is not relevant in and of itself to finance, because a depreciation expense is not a cash flow.

Why does finance place all of its emphasis on cash flows? Because finance focuses on the organization's ability to command resources (goods and services) and capital and its ability to *service its capital* in the future. At root, these abilities rely directly on the use of cash, of money.

Money is a resource like any other, in that an organization must pay for the privilege of using it. Examples include paying interest on a loan or on a bond issue (debt financing), distributing profits (dividends) to partners (stockholders) for profit (equity financing), or providing charity care and supporting teaching and research (not-for-profit equity financing). The organization's ability to make such "rent" payments, plus its ability to repatriate the capital itself directly, affects whether or not it will be able to attract new capital in the future.

Buying resources and servicing capital ultimately requires cash. You cannot meet next Friday's payroll with accounts receivable, revenue, or even income

---

[8] If the supplies were paid for at an earlier time, finance would have noted the outlay at that time; if the supplies are not yet paid for, a debt (liability) has been incurred, and finance will recognize the future outlay as a reduction of debt.

(all accounting measures). You can only meet the payroll with cash or its equivalent, e.g., checks drawn against bank balances. This is why decision making, analysis, and evaluation in finance look at the ability of the organization to meet next Friday's payroll, to buy supplies next month, to service its capital into the indefinite future, i.e., to generate required levels of cash flow. You can defer some things in the short term by borrowing money, of course, but ultimately you must have the cash to repay the borrowing. Thus, while you can shift future cash flows around in time, at some point you finally get to the economic bottom line requiring cash in the bank.

In identifying organizational cash flows, finance focuses on *incremental analysis*, because it is analyzing the future for the specific purpose of assisting managers in making decisions. That is, finance considers only changes in cash flows that may result from a decision. Should we buy a new computer for the accounting department? Finance analysis will look at the timing and amount of cash outflows and inflows only to the extent that they differ from what they might be if the new computer is not purchased.

In finance, the time value of money is always explicit. A dollar today is always different from a dollar tomorrow. If you try to add a January dollar to a December dollar, you are doing what your second grade teacher told you never to do; you are adding apples and oranges. From an economic point of view, January and December dollars are not the same thing, partly because the effect of inflation causes their purchasing power to differ. They are also not the same thing for a variety of other reasons having nothing whatsoever to do with purchasing power. Even if a dollar in January bought the same quantity of real goods and services as a dollar would in December, (i.e., there was no inflation or deflation), you would not be indifferent to the choice between these two dollars at different points in time. If you receive a choice between a 1986 dollar's worth of purchasing power today and a 1986 dollar's worth of purchasing power a year from now, you would still choose the dollar today rather than the purchasing-power-adjusted dollar a year from today. If nothing else, you could always take the dollar today and invest it at a risk-free real (after-inflation) investment rate of two or three percent. That two or three percent represents the compensation required to induce people to defer consumption of real resources.

The finance function includes (1) constructing sophisticated forecasts of distinct uncertain and risky sets of future cash flows, each associated with alternative courses of organizational action; (2) establishing valuation criteria based on estimates of required rates of return[9]; (3) using those criteria to evaluate the relative worth of alternative sets of cash flow streams; and (4) assisting managers in integrating this economic information into decision-making and planning processes.

---

[9] Organizations must service their capital to include paying "rent" on the money/resources they use in providing their health care service or product. But how much rent must be paid? Capital suppliers (whether debt or equity) will require a certain **rate of return** on their funds. In an analogous manner, the organization must also achieve a certain rate of return when it allocates these capital resources to one use or another. Thus, finance has as one of its most basic and important functions ascertaining the appropriate rates of return an organization must (on average) attain from the goods and services it provides in order to achieve long-run economic survival.

Finance forecasts and evaluations are primarily designed for internal, managerial purposes rather than for outside parties, and they are not to be relied upon for external applications or as a vehicle for the implementation of public policy as are the outputs of accounting; they are an input to decision-making and planning processes, primarily internal.

There are several broad categories of decisions that are amenable to analysis from a finance perspective. These include (1) decisions focused on near-term cash flows, so-called "working capital management," (2) capital structure decisions, (3) capital acquisition and disbursement decisions, and 4) long-term investment/divestment choices, so-called "capital budgeting" decisions.

Management of the organization's near-term cash inflows and outflows addresses questions such as, "How much cash should we keep in the bank?" "How big should our inventories be?" "What should our policy be on charging interest on past due accounts?" "What's our collection policy?" "How fast should we pay our bills?" "Should we invest in Treasury bills?" "Should we prepay insurance premiums?" Working capital management decisions are generally based on (1) how variable the organization's cash flows are and (2) what effect the choices have on an organization's ability to meet its required rate(s) of return.

Capital structure matters are another decision area to which the health care industry has paid very little attention historically. Very few organizations have explicit policy positions on the mix of debt and equity that finances their assets and programs. For each organization, there is some particular capital structure range that offers optimal cost and risk characteristics, and, typically, that structure *does* include significant quantities of debt and/or lease financing.

Capital acquisition and disbursement decisions address the raising and servicing of capital. This is different from the capital structure decision, which concerns the *proportions* of debt and equity capital used by an organization. Capital acquisition, by contrast, deals with how you plan to bring capital into the organization as cash (or, in the case of leasing, as real assets). Capital disbursement involves planning for what goes back out the door as cash or in-kind dividend payments, salary "bonuses" to owners, other distributions of accounting income, and interest and principal payments on debt. For debt capital, should we have level debt service, balloon payments, declining debt service? For equity capital, how much should we retain, how much should we repatriate? Correctly structured, these types of transactions ensure organizational continuity, both in being able to provide health services and in having needed access to the capital markets.

The so-called "capital budgeting decision"[10] encompasses all decisions involving the initiation and/or abandonment of programs and services and the resultant retention and/or termination of personnel. Should we acquire this equipment,

---

[10] This is an inappropriate label, since the subject matter in this decision catagory involves neither capital nor budgeting.

initiate this new service, hire this physician, sell off this part of the business, close this department, not replace persons at retirement? How do we structure a portfolio of assets, people, and programs?

In all four categories of decisions just described, finance provides the economic component, the projection of what will best enable the organization to meet or exceed its capital supplier's required rates of return, thereby preserving or enhancing organizational *value*. That is what finance is all about.

The Changing Role of the Chief Financial Officer

As recently as the 1960s,, the health care industry had very little competent financial management. Indeed, the state of fiscal management within most health care provider organizations, if it existed at all, was roughly comparable to the level of fiscal sophistication in the rest of American industry in the 1870s. In prior decades, when most health care providers in the private sector were largely supported by philanthropy and public-sector grants, and when health care costs were not an item of major national policy concern, fiscal management beyond simple bookkeeping and occasional audits was seen largely as a luxury.

It is really only since the advent of the major national entitlement programs, Medicare and Medicaid, that the majority of health care providers has instituted double-entry accrual accounting. In the years since 1965, the health care industry has developed highly competent financial accounting, and, since the advent of Medicare's Prospective Payment System and the rise of prepaid health care, has added some of the most sophisticated cost accounting found in any domestic industry. In addition to financial accounting and cost accounting, increasing use of managerial accounting, especially in the areas of budgeting and control, is also occurring. What is only now emerging, however, is the adoption of the finance techniques that have recently been the subject of Nobel prizes and have been at the forefront of fiscal management for the rest of American industry since shortly after World War II.

Thus, while today's CFO is light years away from the green-eyeshade bookkeeper who ran the business office of the 1940s and 1950s, he or she is much more likely to use a cost accounting approach to pricing than one involving net present value (a finance method discussed later in this chapter) and much more likely to rely on balance sheet information on organizational value than to build alternative systems to estimate market values directly. The key to sound fiscal management is to appreciate the strengths and weaknesses of all of these approaches to resource allocation, to appreciate the interrelationships between fiscal and nonfiscal elements within an organization,and to be able to communicate broadly within the organization, speaking not in "fiscal" tongues but in common language.

Value: Measurement, Maintenance, Enhancement
This section introduces the following concepts of finance:

✦ Debt and Equity Capital
✦ Rate of Return
  — "Pure" interest or "the time value of money"
  — Adjustment for expected inflation
  — Business risk
  — Adjustment for taxation
  — Interest rate risk
✦ Financial Risk and Capital Structure
✦ Cost of Capital and Weighted Average Cost of Capital
✦ Net Present Value

These concepts and the techniques related to them form the foundations for financial evaluation. They are used to evaluate an organization's current financial status and to evaluate what effect, if any, a given proposal or course of action will have on that financial status. The underlying normative principle of finance is that each discrete organizational activity should at least "pay for itself," because, if too many activities are "losers" (without offsetting "winners"), the organization will eventually find its survival threatened. Finance is also quite pragmatic and recognizes that there are times when activities should be supported even though they are not fiscally viable by themselves, if the organization is capable of providing that support. For example, professional personnel might be encouraged to teach at local universities or do research in clinical areas. For these purposes, they receive release time or its equivalent. From a financial perspective, this policy has a direct, measurable cost and no associated measurable income. Yet there is little doubt that having participation in such activities benefits the organization's reputation.

The point is that finance always focuses on the measurable economic consequences of an organization's actions. This analysis is, of course, only one input, though certainly a very important one, into the organization's decision-making and planning processes.

Debt and Equity Capital
The economic foundation of any for-profit or not-for-profit private-sector organization (in the health care field or in any other industry) is its capital. That capital, whatever its mix of debt and equity, supports the entire structure of assets owned (or resources controlled) and programs engaged in by the organization. The ultimate success, indeed the very survival, of the organization depends on the extent to which its utilization of assets and program activities provides fiscal returns sufficient to preserve and/or enhance the underlying capital base.

Preserving and enhancing capital is a fundamental task of any organization in the private sector. Within the private sector, of course, we have both for-profit and not-for-profit organizations. We may characterize not-for-profit organizations as entities that should, at minimum, preserve (maintain) the economic value of their capital, while for-profit organizations need to go the further step of enhancing the economic value of their capital.

For-profit organizations are created to increase the wealth of their owners. This can happen in two ways. First, economic profits can be returned to the owners in cash. Second, such profits can be reinvested in the organization, which increases the market value of owner's equity. In accounting terms, equity is literally the extent to which the value of all organizational assets exceeds the value of all organizational liabilities (debts). In the real (financial) world, the owners' equity is the market value of the owners' claim on the organization if they were to try to sell those claims.

In the not-for-profit case, the "owners" are considered to be the community or the public at large. The return to the community is the services that the organization provides and its ability to continue to provide those services over time. As good stewards, managers of not-for-profit organizations must also attempt to make an accounting profit (i.e., to have revenues exceed expenses).[11] But how large a profit and what the organization does with it are entirely different questions. For example, a not-for-profit provider having a "profit" in a given year might choose to use the portion that a for-profit counterpart might use for dividends or owner wealth enhancing investment to (1) lower its charges (or, given current history, simply hold them constant while competitors' rates go up); (2) offer additional services in nonincome-producing areas such as health education, support of research, or additional charity or deeply discounted care; (3) retain and invest monies in relatively liquid, low-risk assets, helping to carry the organization through lean times; or (4) replace or add real assets to improve the quality of or access to services provided.

The key concept here is that all organizations must make an affirmative accounting profit (have revenues greater than expenses) if they are to survive in the long run. This is equally true of not-for-profit and for-profit firms. What distinguishes the two is what is done with the profit, if any, that exceeds the amount needed to preserve capital.

Preservation of Capital

The term "preservation of capital" has a very specific economic meaning. What we wish to preserve or maintain is the *real value* of capital, the claims of the existing suppliers of the fiscal resources supporting the activities of our organization. Because capital comes to us from an external, competitive marketplace,

---

[11] To illustrate why a "zero bottom line" on an income statement is unacceptable, indeed why a small positive bottom line may also be inadequate, consider the following: If your investment advisor had you invest $100,000 on January 1 for one year and you received a check the following December 31 for $102,000 for the full liquidation of your investment, you would have a $2,000 bottom line, a $2,000 accounting profit (and if you were a taxable entity, you would owe income taxes on that $2,000). You would also be looking for a new investment advisor, because notwithstanding your "profitable" year, you are less wealthy at December 31 than you were the previous January 1, because, if for no other reason, $102,000 will buy less December 31 than 100,000 would have a year earlier.

our ability to satisfy those who have, in the past, supplied us with capital is the key element to our being able to attract new supplies of capital from those or other suppliers in the future.

Satisfying capital suppliers means meeting their expectations. All suppliers of capital to the private sector expect some form of return in exchange for their having supplied the capital, and those expectations exist whether the capital was supplied to a for-profit or a not-for-profit organization.

Suppliers of *debt capital* are readily identified as institutions and individuals having contractual claims against the organization (i.e., formal, written expectation), for example, a commercial bank that has extended credit, an insurance company holding a mortgage note, a pension fund holding a private placement of bonds, or individuals holding bonds that were publicly offered. The expectations of suppliers of debt capital as to returns are clear and explicit. They are embodied in the contractual terms agreed to in advance by themselves and the borrowing organization in a loan agreement, mortgage contract, bond indenture, or whatever.

Most suppliers of *equity capital* to a for-profit organization are clearly identifiable. Shareholders of a corporation, the partners in a partnership, or the owner of a sole proprietorship supply equity capital to those organizations. For the not-for-profit health care provider, equity suppliers are somewhat more diverse and, generally, much more difficult to identify individually. The list may include private donors of cash, be they major philanthropists, private foundations, or persons contributing a few dollars to an annual fund drive; volunteers who provide wage and salary expense relief to the institution or program; payers of tax monies that flow through a governmental entity to the provider by grant, appropriation, or designation[12]; and a small number of recipients of health services who, themselves or via third parties, pay more than the economic cost for those services. Because of the breadth and diversity of these equity capital suppliers, we generally refer to them as "society," "the community," or "the service area."

There is, of course, no written contract concerning specific returns to suppliers of common equity capital. As a result, managers (even of for-profit firms) sometimes fall into the trap of viewing equity capital as a free good, as having no explicit cost—that is, requiring no returns. Nothing could be further from economic reality.

The shareholders or partners of a for-profit organization have very clear expectations of dividends or cash distributions and/or appreciation in the market price of their ownership claim. Suppliers of equity capital to not-for-profit organizations also have specific expectations of return. The fact that these returns are not

---

[12] In addition to direct subsidies, there are indirect subsidies as, for example, the granting of tax-exempt status and the right to issue tax-exempt securities, both of which tend to raise others' taxes and to make up for the governmental revenue shortfalls ("tax expenditures") thus created. Another indirect subsidy is the income-tax deductibility of contributions to 501(c)(3) organizations.

permitted to be in the form of cash distributions or market value appreciation in no way lessens the strength of the expectations or reduces the economic burden on management to meet those expectations. Suppliers of equity capital to not-for-profit health care providers expect those organizations to remain viable into the indefinite future[13]; they expect the social value of the services provided by such organizations to exceed the organizations' charges for providing those services; they expect such organizations to support, as appropriate, relevant educational programs and research; they expect reasonable levels of free and/or discounted care to be provided to certain segments of the community served. Indeed, the range of equity supplier expectations may be quite large.

Required Rate of Return
The rate of return required by any supplier of capital will, of course, vary through time. This is because a generic rate of return conceptually includes compensation for five major factors, any one of which can change at any time in a dynamic marketplace: (1) the pure "time value of money," (2) inflation (deflation), (3) default, (4) untimely/forced liquidation, and (5) expected taxation.

The pure time value of money is simply economic recognition of that (1) consumption of goods and services has positive value to human beings and (2) consumption cannot be postponed indefinitely because of the finite life span of human beings. Individuals, directly and through the organizations they form, draw satisfaction from consumption[14] and require compensation for anything that delays that consumption. That is, because we prefer to consume sooner rather than later and because supplying capital to others effectively delays the supplier's ability to use those funds for consumption, a "pure rate of interest" is required to compensate for the delay. Empirically, the pure rate of interest as an annual rate has been in the 2-3 percent range.

For example, suppose a bank supplies $36,000 of capital to an organization today and expects the loan to be paid back after one year. The bank may require (expect) $900 (2½ percent) worth of compensation one year from now in recognition of the fact that the bank's money has been tied up for one year. Thus, a payment to the bank of $36,900 one year hence would provide a full return *of* and *on* capital.[15]

The second component of a required rate of return is the additional compensation necessary in an inflationary environment to compensate the capital supplier for expected loss of purchasing power. (In the case of expected deflation, an

---

[13] The accountant embodies this expectation in applying the "ongoing enterprise" principle; the attorney does the same thing in referring to the corporation as "an infinite-life individual" under the law.

[14] Consumption is broadly defined here to encompass not only the acquisition of services and material goods, but also charitable activity from which the donor derives satisfaction.

[15] Return **of** capital is exactly what it sounds like: the organization pays back money it has been supplied. This is the case when we pay off the **principle** portion of the loan. Return **on** capital is the "rent" paid for the use of the money, as, for example, the interest portion of a loan payment. The **combination** of returns of and on capital is called the return **to** capital.

adjustment *reducing* the overall required rate of return would occur.) Between the time the capital is initially supplied and the time(s) that returns to capital are made, price increases in the capital supplier's "market basket" of goods and services will have reduced the real value of the supplier's initial investment. The purchasing power adjustment that compensates for this expected loss of value is applied both to the initial capital itself and to the compensation-for-delayed-consumption (pure interest) return.

Continuing the numerical example begun above, if a 6 percent inflation rate is expected (that is, it will take $10.60 one year from now to buy the same quantities of goods and services now costing $10.00), the bank would require certain (guaranteed) returns worth $39,114 one year hence ($36,900 plus 6 percent of $36,900).

The third component of an overall required rate of return on capital is compensation for the risk of possible nonpayment or delay in payment of some or all of the total return due to the capital supplier.[16] Default arises because of an insufficiency of cash to service capital, reflecting cash flow variability that derives primarily from an organization's basic economic activity (business risk), and for each class of capital supplier can be mitigated or magnified by the relative position (priority or lack thereof) of that class's claim among all capital claims on the organization (financial risk).[17] Financial risk and its implications will be considered in more detail in the next section. Business risk arises from the nature of the economic environment and from operational characteristics of each organization. One way to think about business risk is by arraying three categories of elements: *systemic risk* (inter- and intrasystem phenomena, e.g., political factors such as expropriation or nationalization of assets, fluctuations in exchange rates, monetary and fiscal policy), *market risk* (e.g., elements of competition, public and/or private regulation, supplier power, technological obsolescence), and *organizational risk* (e.g., quality of managerial and operating personnel and processes, input/output efficiency). All of these elements interacting will cause some organizations to experience cash flows that fall short of what is required to meet the expectations of some or all of their capital suppliers, with a resultant default.

Continuing our example, suppose that the bank expects a four percent complete default rate (i.e., for every 100 loans of this type made, 96 are paid in full on time, and 4 go to total default and repay nothing). To cover this contingency, the bank will charge a premium on each loan it makes. To compute the premium, divide the total payment that fully compensates the bank for the pure time value of money and for inflation by one minus the failure rate:

$$\$39,114/(1-.04) = \$39,114/.96 = \$40,473.75$$

---

[16] The so-called "risk-free rate" which is the required rate of return on federal government treasury securities is a rate which contemplates no risk of default. This is because the federal government literally can't default since the government could always manufacture the stuff (money) that its securities promise to pay. The risk-free rate, however, recognizes that such securities have all of the other four components of risk that require compensation.

[17] E.g., employees get paid before suppliers, suppliers get paid before bondholders, secured debt gets paid off before unsecured debt, debt gets paid off before equity holders.

This assures the bank of full returns on all of its loans by spreading the risk of failure across all the loans it makes:

$$96 \times \$40,473.75 = \$3,911,400$$

$$100 \times \$39,114.00 = \$3,911,400$$

Other, slightly more complicated calculations are possible that would take into account partial repayments and late repayments.

The fourth component of a basic rate of return deals with the generic risks associated with an uncertain future. Suppliers of capital, like all managers, attempt to forecast future economic conditions. Good as our crystal balls and computer models may be, no one can have absolute confidence in forecasts of next year's monetary policy, inflation rate, and rates of taxation or of the likelihood of default on a claim. Thus, required rates of return fluctuate daily, as expectations about future events and conditions change. In this fluctuating environment, the capital supplier bears the risks associated with the possible necessity of having to sell the capital claim for an unknown price[18] to someone else prior to its original or expected maturity. The further in the future the expected maturity, the greater is the possibility of having to do this. Not only is there the possibility of sustaining a capital loss, but generally there will also be conversion or transaction costs associated with the untimely or forced liquidation of the claim.

These risks of loss are in part related to the amount of time remaining until all returns to a capital claim are expected to be realized—the longer the time, the greater the risk—but are also related to the natural degree of volatility in the claim-specific risk factors noted above, and the efficiency or lack thereof in the secondary market for the claim. Typically, an additional premium for bearing such risks, an "illiquidity premium"[19] is observable in required rates of return as compensation for future interest rate (and capital value) fluctuation. While there is no way to calculate an exact amount for the illiquidity premium, it might be as little as one percent for a one-year maturity and several percentage points for a 10-year maturity.

In our example, rather than requiring $40,743.75, the bank might ask for an additional $404.25 (a bit less than one percent), or a total of $41,148.

The fifth component of marketplace required rates of return is compensation for taxation. Different taxes may be levied simultaneously by several different levels of government, and the nature and rate of taxation levied by each may depend on the characteristics of both the supplier of the capital and the user of the capital.

---

[18] Or even a known price in the case of a discretionary call or a random mandatory call by the organization to which the capital was supplied.

[19] One sometimes hears the term "liquidity premium." This refers to the higher price the market typically (but not always) places on claims with shirt-term maturities. Since prices and rates of return are inversely related, the terms "illiquidity premium" or "duration premium" refer to the usually higher **rates** (lower prices) on longer time-to-maturity claims.

Suppose, for our example, that the return *on* the $36,000 in capital (that is, all return in excess of $36,000, or $5,148, is considered taxable income. Because that $5,148 is seen as what is necessary to fairly compensate the capital supplier for real interest, inflation, the risk of default, and the risk of untimely liquidation, the capital supplier must receive before-tax compensation of sufficient magnitude so that after meeting the attendant tax liability, $5,148 will remain. To find the appropriate before-tax amount, simply divide the required after-tax dollar return on capital by one minus the applicable marginal tax rate. If the bank in this example had to pay tax at a marginal rate of 20 percent,[20] the required payment would be:

$$\$36,000 + \$5,148/(1-.20) = \$36,000 + \$5,148/0.80 = \$36,000 + 6,435 =$$
$$\$42,435, \text{ or a } 17.875\% \text{ required rate of return}$$

The capital marketplace brings together suppliers and users of capital representing the full spectrum of different tax and inflation environments, all manner of sensitivities to risks, as well as widely divergent opinions as to future economic conditions and business risks. Hence, market-determined rates of return ultimately represent the relative supplies of and demands for capital from many heterogeneous market participants. Nonetheless, market clearing rates of return necessarily satisfy capital suppliers in the conceptual dimensions noted. If they did not, the capital would not be supplied.

Classes of Capital Suppliers, Financial Risk, and Required Rates
The discussion above of required rates of return was generic for all suppliers of capital and mentioned only in footnote 13 certain distinctions among various suppliers of capital. Complex capital structures may contain several types of debt, a number of categories of equity, and various forms of leasing. For our purposes here, however, we will consider only the simplest case—that in which we have only two kinds of suppliers of capital, both internally homogeneous: suppliers of equity capital and suppliers of debt capital.

Although debt suppliers may not have been the first parties chronologically to provide capital to the organization, they are definitely the parties first in line to receive returns to capital. This is because organizations enter into explicit contracts with suppliers of debt, promising to pay them specific sums of interest and principal at definite future times. These contractual claims take precedence over returns to equity suppliers. That is, in general, debt's contractual claims must be fully satisfied before any equity returns are allowed.

Therefore, debt is always viewed as less risky than equity, because debt has first claim on the organization's cash flows. There is, therefore, a difference in the *financial risk* faced by suppliers of debt and equity capital.

If an organization were 100 percent equity-financed, equity would bear all of the risks and costs discussed earlier. If the organization approached being 100 percent debt-financed, debt would have assumed almost all of these risks and costs. At

---

[20] This assumes that there are no offsetting incremental deductions for expenses. If there were, they would lessen the tax burden.

points in the middle (say 50 percent debt and 50 percent equity), debt's first claim on the organization's resources makes it less risky than equity and thus its required rate of return will be less. Indeed, debt's risk is not only less than equity's, it is less than the average risk of the overall organization.

In a parallel manner, equity's inherent risk would be magnified by the financial risk associated with increasing proportions of debt having a priority claim in the capital structure. As debt claims a greater and greater share of the operational cash flows available to service capital, it becomes increasingly likely that variability in those flows might leave little or no funds after debt service to meet the expectations of equity suppliers. Equity suppliers require a higher rate of return to compensate them for bearing this financial risk over and above the other risks and costs. If there is any debt at all, equity's required rate of return will be higher than debt's *and* higher than the average rate of return for the overall organization. At high levels of debt financing, equity holders might well require rates of return in the 30-40 percent per annum range.

The Cost of Capital

Up to this point, required rates of return have been discussed primarily from the perspective of the capital supplier. The other side of the coin, of course, is the *cost of capital* to the user. In the simplest of cases, these are identical. What the capital supplier receives is what it costs the organization. Various circumstances, however, can change that identity and cause the cost of debt service to the organization to be less than the required rate of return actually received by the capital supplier.

For example, a corporate for-profit provider pays tax on its net income, taxable revenues less deductible expenses. Interest paid is one deductible expense. Therefore, an organization paying taxes at a rate of 40 percent and paying lenders 10 percent interest has a real (after-tax) cost of only 6 percent (1 - 0.4 = 0.6; 0.6 x 10% = 6%). The capital supplier still gets 10%, but 4% of that is, in effect, a governmental subsidy. Another example is the fact that for-profit and not-for-profit hospitals may be subject to Medicare capital cost passthroughs and/or still receive some cost-based reimbursement during the 1990s. Because interest is an allowable cost for these purposes and results in greater reimbursement than if returns on capital were associated with equity rather than debt, the economic effect is the same as the income tax effect; it lowers the net cost of debt to the organization, because a third party is, in effect, subsidizing a portion of the return actually received by the capital supplier.[21]

Provider and payment differences aside, however, the basic point is that the economics of producing the returns to capital (the costs of capital) need to be distinguished from the returns themselves (as viewed by the capital suppliers receiving them).

---

[21] It is also possible to have a lower cost of capital in other ways. For example, a nonprofit provider may be also able to pay interest that is nontaxable to the lender, thereby lowering its cost of capital by choice of financing vehicle. (Tax-free bonds are the most common example of this type of arrangement.) This mechanism, however, does not cause a difference between the organization's cost of capital and the capital supplier's required rate of return since it simply lowers both.

The long-run survival of any private sector organization, for-profit or not-for-profit, depends on its ability to renew existing capital (not assets) and to attract new capital from time to time. This ability to succeed in attracting infusions of capital from an increasingly competitive capital market relates specifically to the organization's demonstrated ability to preserve the real economic value of existing capital. That value is preserved only if each class of capital supplier receives its respective required rate of return. Because parts of that required rate of return may be provided (or reduced by external parties (e.g., taxation or reimbursement authorities), internal organizational decisions need focus only on the net cost of capital. Thus, a provider's operational fiscal returns must attain the cost of capital threshold, so that, when supplemented (or reduced) by external parties, capital suppliers will receive their required rates of return and be willing to renew or expand their provision of capital to the organization.

Meeting the expectations of some but not all capital suppliers is insufficient. For example, paying all of the contractual interest and principal payments on time is not, by itself, enough to guarantee future access to capital. It is also necessary to preserve the value of equity capital in order to maintain a strong overall capital structure. A weak equity position is just as surely a hindrance to future borrowing as is failure to meet debt service payments.

Selection of Organization Activities

The "bottom line" (both figuratively and literally) of financial analysis is determining whether or not a given organizational activity (e.g., opening a new clinic, adding more physicians, buying a computer, adding a new service) will pay for itself in the long run or be a drain on the organization's resources (i.e., equity). To do this, finance computes the *weighted average cost of capital*, identifies the *incremental operational cash flows* associated with the activity, and, from them, determines the *net present value* of the alternative or activity.

An organization obtains capital from many different sources: bank loans, individual investors or contributors, grants, bond issues, etc. Each source will have an associated cost of capital. One useful statistic for financial analysis, therefore, is the "weighted average cost of capital" (WACC). This is simply the cost of capital for each supplier weighted by its proportion of total capital measured at market value. For example, suppose a provider has total capital of $1,000,000[22]: a $250,000 loan and a tax-exempt bond issue for $500,000 at net (after-tax and after-reimbursement) costs of 10 percent and 7 percent, respectively, and a $250,000 grant from the government at a presumed equity rate of 12 percent. The WACC of this organization would be:

$$\underset{\text{(Loan)}}{\frac{250{,}000}{1{,}000{,}000}} \times .10 + \underset{\text{(Bond)}}{\frac{500{,}000}{1{,}000{,}000}} \times .07 + \underset{\text{(Grant)}}{\frac{250{,}000}{1{,}000{,}000}} \times .12 = \underset{\text{(WACC)}}{9.00\%}$$

---

[22] In WACC computations, market values of debt and equity claims are always used rather than "book" or accounting values.

Second, the incremental, operational cash flows associated with the activity must be identified. Operational cash flows are nonaccrual measures of all the cash flows in and out of the organization *other than* (1) cash flows to and from capital suppliers (e.g., interest payments) and (2) cash flows triggered by capital supplier flows (e.g., tax reductions or extra reimbursement in recognition of interest payments). Operational cash flows, therefore, exclude contributions and dividends, but include inflows from asset liquidation and outflows for asset acquisition.

In addition to the requirement that cash flows be of the operational rather than the capital type, they also must be strictly incremental. This simply means that we count only those cash flows that will change as a result of the decision regarding the proposal under consideration.[23]

The fiscal evaluation of any proposal begins with an estimate of the expected incremental operational cash flows associated with the proposal, period by period, over an appropriate future time. Once this stream of cash flows is obtained, it must be evaluated relative to the organization's WACC. This is because organizations should focus on their cost of capital rather than on capital's required rate of return. Specifically, the WACC is used as the "rate of discount" with which to find the value today of a proposal's expected incremental future operational cash flows (including the proposal's expected investment outlays now and henceforth). This value today is called the proposal's net present value (NPV). A positive NPV means that a proposal pays for itself (including the cost of capital to support it) and that there will be funds left over that can be put to other uses. An NPV of zero means that a proposal breaks even in economic terms—it will pay for itself but generate no additional resources beyond the required returns. A negative NPV means that the organization will have to subsidize the proposal, because it cannot be economically self-supporting.[24]

Calculating a proposal's NPV using the WACC as the discount rate involves determining the relative value of each of the incremental operational cash flows occurring at different times.

---

[23] One circumstance to be careful of is when the adoption of a proposal obviates a future operational cash flow otherwise required in the absence of favorable consideration afforded the proposal under consideration. For example, suppose a room would need to be repainted next year. A proposal to initiate a new service this year calls for the complete renovation of this space now, dispensing with the cost of repainting the room next year. For the purpose of analyzing the proposal, the cost of painting the room next year is treated as a relevant, incremental, operational cash **inflow** next year associated with the new service proposal. This is because the proposal saves money that would otherwise have been spent.

[24] Note that a proposal that generates positive net income as measured by GAAP may have a negative NVP. For example, suppose you invest $100,000 for one year and at the end of the year receive back $102,500, a 2 ½% rate of return. We can presume that you will not be a happy investor since almost certainly $102,500 will not command as many real resources at the end of the year at the $100,000 would have at the beginning of the year, if only because of inflation (and you will have received nothing in compensation for the delay in consumption or the bearing of risk during the year). Nonetheless, your investment is profitable for the year and under GAAP you have $2,500 of positive income. And to add injury to the injury, if you are a taxable entity, that $2,500 will also subject you to and income tax liability. Positive accounting income is not necessarily good news.

For all the reasons discussed earlier, as long as there is a positive rate of return, a dollar in hand today is more valuable than a dollar expected tomorrow. If a 20 percent per annum rate of return is required (or available), one dollar invested today at that rate will be worth $1.20 one year hence. Similarly, one dollar expected a year from now is worth only 83 ⅓ cents today.[25] The discount factor (1.20 in these examples) is equal to one plus the appropriate discount rate expressed as a decimal.

Because the calculation of an NPV is largely mechanical,[26] we won't go into great detail here, but a simplified numerical example in Appendix E to this chapter illustrates the application of this concept of value measurement.

Net present value is a powerful concept that allows comparison of different courses of action and their consequences in economic terms. However, it is important to remember that financial evaluation is just one input into the overall decision making process.

Some Normative Considerations

Positive-NPV activities increase an organization's value (i.e., the value of its equity) even after having satisfied all suppliers of capital, including equity. The increase in value in today's dollars is equal to the positive amount of NPV. Negative-NPV activities show the amount by which the value of the organization will decline in today's dollars if all required rates of return are still met. (Meeting such requirements is accomplished by drawing down the value of existing equity, a process in which many providers engage, often unknowingly.) In the long term, of course, organizations with negative-NPV portfolios cease to exist through one of two mechanisms. In the most severe case, termination by bankruptcy occurs. In the milder circumstance, future access to the capital markets is denied and a less traumatic liquidation or sale or merger occurs.

For-profit providers have an economic obligation to maximize the wealth of their ownership, subject to all the usual legal and ethical constraints. Hence, for-profit providers should actively seek as many positive-NPV activities in their portfolio of assets and programs as possible.

By contrast, not-for-profit providers should be seen as an overall neutral-NPV portfolio of activities. This in no way precludes the growth of the organization, for it says nothing about the number or size of activities engaged in. Rather, the "rule" is that not-for-profit organizations should seek an overall portfolio of activities that achieves only a small positive-NPV, meeting the required rates of return of all capital suppliers and relevant community constituencies.

For example, consider the example of a hospital or a clinic that is considering a

---

[25] $0.83 ⅓ return of capital plus $0.16 ⅔ return on capital (20% of $0.83 ⅓) equals a $1.00 total return.

[26] Many pocket calculators are preprogrammed to perform present value calculations and routine business software packages include such programs. In addition, tables are available to aid in the hand calculation of present value.

new marketing program that (it is predicted) will have a highly positive NPV. A for-profit organization might choose to increase dividends or distributions to equity as the new income is realized, or it might choose to reinvest the "extra" dollars in activities that increase owners' equity. A not-for-profit organization is faced with the same question: What do we do with the extra dollars? It might choose to add a health education program (return of social value to community); support clinical research or teaching (return to community) and probably an "in-kind" or noncash bonus to workers (increasing the organization's viability); reduce prices to some patients or provide additional charity care (social dividend); or simply retain the money as liquid, short-term assets, such as CDs or T-bills (increase organization viability).

A negative-NPV proposal, by definition, is incapable of sustaining itself economically. Assuming all possible cost efficiencies have been incorporated in the proposal, the only way to adjust the value of such a proposal upward is to increase its operational cash inflows by posting higher prices (rates). If, ultimately, such increases are constrained by competition, rate regulation, ordinary price elasticity in the marketplace, or other economic or political factors, and the NPV still remains negative, the proposal must be rejected as a "mainframe"[27] activity. However, this does not necessarily mean that the proposal should be rejected totally. Financial analysis using NPV is only one input into overall decision making. Besides economic factors, there are two other generic concerns that must be examined: long-run strategic payoffs and "social" value.

At this point, the organization's board should review such uneconomic proposals (assuming they are of sufficient magnitude to warrant this). The substance of the proposal (e.g., the actual service to be delivered) may be viewed by the board as so important to the community that the board will declare the activity a dividend (to the community)[28] or so integrally intertwined with the organization's mission that it is considered essential. Neither step should be taken lightly (which, of course, is why the matter should be brought to the board in the first place).

Take the case of a social dividend to the community. If the provider is currently meeting the expectations of its equity capital suppliers, does not offset the new dividend by a reduction in an existing dividend, and wishes to maintain the current value of its capital (i.e., does not wish to partially liquidate through a return of capital), the board, by declaring the dividend, is saying the community expects (requires) the dividend as part of its overall return. This simply means

---

[27] A "mainframe" activity is one that is economically self-supporting, "a tub on its own bottom" not requiring external or cross-subsidization to exist. Mainframe activities are those meeting the WACC criterion, thereby providing the cash flows needed to service the organization's capital.

[28] Depending on corporate philosophy, for-profit as well as non-profit providers may choose widely different approaches to community dividends. The nonprofit "community-owned" provider, of course, has a much more direct economic tie to its service area, and typically must meet higher expectations regarding returns to equity capital in the form of in-kind dividends than the for-profit provider which also returns cash to the "community" in the form of taxes.

that unless new inflows of equity capital can be found, mainframe (nondividend) activities will have to bear the additional cost of the new dividend, thereby implying price increases.

If the cash inflows from existing mainframe activities cannot be increased (again assuming cost efficiency has already been attained), and new equity capital is not forthcoming, the dividend that has been declared is, in effect, a partial liquidating dividend. There is absolutely nothing wrong with declaring a partial liquidating dividend, of course, as long as it is done consciously, explicitly. Adopting negative-NPV projects (effective dividends) without being aware of their long-run economic implications, however, can clearly endanger long-run organizational survival.

With respect to strategic decisions to invest in "essential" activities, it is important that organizational decision making and board policy formulation take a long-run perspective if the organization is to remain viable in a dynamic and competitive environment. On the other hand, the factors cited above (cross-subsidization and partial liquidation of capital) also need to be considered. This approach to explicit, board-level formulation of dividend policy has the major advantage of bringing issues of cross-subsidization out of the shadows and placing them on top of the table for direct deliberation and decision making.

Finally, all organizations should attempt to minimize their WACC. For a given set of programs and activities, a lower WACC will clearly generate more wealth for for-profit ownership and greater price reductions in the not-for-profit sector. Additionally, more proposals will have NPVs greater than or equal to zero, thereby allowing a broader range of both mainframe services and dividends.

Techniques for minimizing the WACC are among a number of advanced fiscal management subjects that cannot be addressed in detail here, but they would include determining and implementing an optimal capital structure, taking a wide variety of possible actions to minimize perceived business risk, and ensuring that the lowest cost sources of capital are being tapped. It is worth noting that the latter technique is one of the stronger economic arguments for retaining tax-exempt debt financing for not-for-profit providers. The lower WACC that results from tax-exempt financing also permits the broader range of mainframe services and dividends noted above.

Further Study of Finance and Accounting

As we have seen above, finance and accounting are important functional areas within the discipline of management.

Finance is primarily concerned with assisting managers in making resource allocation and financing decisions that are consistent with economic value criteria. Finance focuses on forecasting future fiscal events and on evaluating alternative forecasts against value criteria tailored to each organization. For a fuller appreciation of finance as a managerial discipline, see the Brealey and Gapenski references.

You should exercise caution in assuming a book really deals with finance just because the word "finance" or "financial" is in the title. For example, the Cleverley and Neumann references are excellent treatments of managerial and cost accounting, but they do not deal with any significant amount of finance, even though one might erroneously assume from their titles that they do.

Accounting focuses on ex-post reporting to internal and external parties, on the attribution of long-run resource costs to individual units of output, and on the analysis of such information. These emphases have produced particular process-es and formats through which information is generated, reported, and analyzed. For ex-post reporting, there are income statements, balance sheets, and state-ments of "cash flow" that are generated by double-entry accounting systems applying generally accepted accounting principles. Cost-attribution involves many complex ways of assigning or allocating categories of resource costs. Managerial accounting encompasses a variety of analytical techniques. To be able to appreciate fully such information requires a solid understanding of the rules and processes by which they are produced. That level of understanding is well beyond the scope of this chapter, but excellent starting points for anyone ·wishing to go more deeply into such material are the Anthony (1993), Pratt, and Horngren references.

References

1. American Institute of Certified Public Accountants Health Care Committee. *Audits of providers of health care services prepared by the Health Care Committee and the Health Care Audit and Accounting Guide Task Force: including statement of position issued by the Accounting Standards Division.* New York: American Institute of Certified Public Accountants, Inc., 1990.

2. Anthony, R. *A Review of Essentials of Accounting.* 5th Edition. Reading, Mass.: Addison-Wesley, 1993.

3. Anthony, R. *The Management Control Function.* Boston, Mass.: Harvard Business School Press, 1988.

4. Anthony, R., and Graham, W. *Management Control in Nonprofit Organizations.* Homewood, Ill.: Irwin, 1988.

5. Berman, H., and others. *The Financial Management of Hospitals,* 7th ed. Ann Arbor, Mich.: Health Administration Press, 1990.

6. Brealey, R., and Myers, S. *Principles of Corporate Finance,* Fourth Edition. New York, N.Y.: McGraw-Hill, 1991.

7. Broyles, R., and Rosko, M. *Fiscal Management of Healthcare Institutions.* Owings Mills, Md.: National Health Publishing, 1990.

8. Cleverley, W. *Essentials of Health Care Finance,* 3rd ed. Rockville, Md.: Aspen Publishers, 1992.

9. Gapenski, L. *Understanding Health Care Finance Management—Text, Cases, and Models,* Ann Arbor, Mich.: Health Administration Press, 1993.

10. Horngren, C., and Foster, G. *Cost Accounting: A Managerial Emphasis,* 7th ed. Englewood Cliffs, N.J.: PrenticeHall, 1991.

11. Kaplan, R. Advanced Management Accounting. Englewood Cliffs, N.J.: PrenticeHall, 1982.

12. Magee, R. *Advanced Managerial Accounting.* Somerset, N.J.: John Wiley & Sons, 1986.

13. Neumann, B., and others. *Financial Management: Concepts and Applications for Health Care Providers,* 2nd ed. Dubuque, Iowa: Kendall/Hunt Publishing, 1988.

14. Pratt, J. *Financial Accounting,* 2nd ed. Cincinnati, Ohio: Southwestern Publishers, Inc., 1993.

15. Suver, J., and others. *Cases in Health Care Financial Management.* Ann Arbor, Mich.: Health Administration Press, 1984.

16. Suver, J., and Neumann, B. *Management Accounting for Healthcare Organizations,* 3rd ed. Oak Brook, Ill., Pluribus Press, 1992.

17. Wrightson, C. *HMO Rate Setting & Financial Strategy.* Ann Arbor, Mich. Health Administration Press, 1990.

Appendix A. Financial Statements

The financial statements produced by an accounting system contain information that can be critical in decision-making processes, especially those engaged in by top management and by parties external to the organization. Collectively, the various financial statements present the financial condition of the organization to management, stockholders, lenders, regulators, and other interested parties. Because typically the statements are prepared in accordance with generally accepted accounting principles (GAAP), the information can be analyzed and compared with that of previous years and, in some cases, with similar institutions. A thorough and continuing analysis of the financial statements can highlight potential problem areas and aid in determining corrective action.

Basic Financial Statements

The three primary types of financial statements are the balance sheet, the income statement, and the statement of "cash flow." Each of these statements has particular strengths and weaknesses for determining the financial condition of the organization.

The Balance Sheet

The balance sheet shows the financial position of the organization at a point in time. This can be the end of the year, the end of the month, or any other time desired by the administrator. Its reliability is determined by the accuracy of the accounting information and the appropriateness of generally accepted accounting principles and regulations for the decision being made. The Financial Accounting Standards Board (FASB) and other professional accounting organizations issue guidance through pronouncements and opinions on appropriate accounting practices for presenting fair financial statements. For example, the physical assets of the organization are typically carried at their initial acquisition costs, the amounts carried in inventory and accounts receivable are a function of the accuracy of the record-keeping system and the time selected for the report. Some organizations will use the calendar year as their reporting period. Others may use another fiscal period that is more appropriate in terms of patient services and census. For example, a December 31 cutoff date for the balance sheet may have been selected more as a matter of tradition than because it is a proper time to analyze the financial position. December may typically be a low census month and some other time may be more representative. A typical balance sheet format and types of accounts are shown in figure A-1, page 120.

The components of the balance sheet are typically classified into definite groupings. For example, current assets include assets that are expected to be converted into cash or expenses within the current operating period, or within one year.

Figure A1. Typical Balance Sheet

MEDICAL CENTER
BALANCE SHEET—JUNE 30, 19x2 and 19x1

Assets	19x2	19x1
CURRENT ASSETS:		
Cash and cash equivalents	$391,767	$1,125,628
Accounts receivable, net of allowance for uncollectible accounts and contractual allowances of $3,393,361 in 19x2 and $2,367,641 in 19x1.	8,399,210	7,524,313
Other accounts receivable	477,274	554,433
Reimbursement settlement receivable	72,601	80,668
Inventory of supplies	356,798	373,901
Prepaid expenses	53,251	80,714
Assets whose use is limited that are required for current liabilities	1,624,400	1,689,400
Total Current Assets	11,375,301	11,429,057
ASSETS WHOSE USE IS LIMITED BY BOARD-DESIGNATION		
Cash and cash equivalents	614,423	1,063,749
Short-term investments	6,348,645	2,966,819
Investment in pooled fund	1,842,483	2,551,979
Accrued interest receivable	31,628	10,079
Total assets whose use is limited	8,837,179	6,592,626
Less- current portion	(1,624,400)	(1,689,400)
Net assets whose use is limited	7,212,779	4,903,226
PROPERTY, PLANT AND EQUIPMENT at cost:		
Hospital operations-		
Land and improvements	1,358,809	1,342,397
Buildings and leasehold improvements	16,607,453	15,556,408
Fixed equipment	14,206,950	14,209,592
Movable equipment	10,401,089	9,769,731
Other		
Construction in progress	80,170	768,910
Total property, plant and equipment	42,654,471	41,647,038
Less accumulated depreciation	(19,645,445)	(17,143,693)
Net property, plant and equipment	23,009,026	24,503,345
DEFERRED PROFESSIONAL LIABILITY COSTS	---	164,000
DEFERRED FINANCING COSTS	533,517	587,313
TOTAL ASSETS	$42,130,623	$41,586,941

Liabilities and Fund Balances	19x2	19x1
CURRENT LIABILITIES		
Accounts payable	$2,326,397	$1,953,484
Accrued payroll, payroll taxes and employee benefits	2,000,348	1,900,659
Accrued interest payable	---	40,895
Other current liabilities	385,821	480,596
Reimbursement settlement payable	665,623	521,561
Payable to related division	630,000	---
Current portion of long-term debt	1,624,400	1,689,400
Total current liabilities	7,632,589	6,586,595
OTHER LIABILITIES AND DEFERRED REVENUE:		
Deferred revenue	70,560	72,240
Reserve for professional liability costs (Note 2)	82,000	164,000
Total other liabilities and deferred revenue	152,560	236,240
LONG-TERM DEBT		
Notes payable	13,949,900	16,354,300
Total long-term debt	13,949,900	16,354,300
Less-current portion	(1,624,400)	(1,689,400)
Net long-term debt	12,325,500	14,664,900
COMMITMENTS AND CONTINGENT LIABILITIES (Note 7)		
FUND BALANCES		
General	21,762,926	20,020,776
Restricted	257,048	78,430
Total fund balances	22,019,974	20,099,206
TOTAL LIABILITIES and FUND BALANCES	$42,130,623	$41,586,941

Assets limited as to use are internally restricted funds that have been identified by management for specific uses. The key term is "internally restricted"; the board can change either the amount or the classification. This can be contrasted to externally restricted funds, which require approval of the donor if changes in use are desired by management. Fixed assets are usually physical plant and equipment, which are expected to benefit more than one period. Fixed assets are converted into current expenses through depreciation techniques. The choice of depreciation methods can have a major impact on reported income and tax liability. Intangible assets are generally listed last because they are the least liquid of the assets and because their actual values depend on the provider's staying in business. Examples include deferred financing costs for debt that has been refinanced or attorney fees for reorganizational costs that have been incurred but must be expended over time because of GAAP.

Offsetting the asset accounts are the liabilities and equity accounts of the organization. Liabilities consist of both short-term (current liabilities) and long-term (payable over more than one year) debt. Equity accounts are composed of the initial capital investment of the owners and the earnings retained in the organization from providing services. Equity accounts for not-for-profit organizations are sometimes called fund balances. The amounts reflect what has been retained in the organization after the amounts due to external creditors have been subtracted from the total assets (Total Assets minus Total Debt equals Equity/Net Worth/Fund Balances). Balance sheet accounts are usually considered to be permanent accounts; that is, they do not close at the end of each accounting period.

The Income Statement

The income statement measures the results of providing services over a period of time. It, too, is prepared in accordance with generally accepted accounting principles. The accrual method (matching of revenues and expenses), the depreciation method (straight line, accelerated), and the inventory valuation method can have a decided impact on reported income. Under the accrual method of accounting, and where noncash expenses such as depreciation are included, the income reported on the income statement is not the same as cash; in fact, using this method, it is possible to report high income and still experience a serious cash shortage. (This problem will be discussed in greater detail later in this section.) A typical income statement is shown in figure A-2, page 122.

The major components of the income statement are the revenue accounts and the expenses accounts. The revenue accounts should be segregated by payer categories. The amounts shown as revenues do not include contractual allowances, discounts, and charity care. Only amounts that have been billed to payers will be included. Bad debts or amounts expected not to be collected are included as an expense account instead of a deduction from revenue. Charity care is only shown as a footnote to the summary statements and are no longer shown as a deduction from revenues. Nonpatient service revenues are shown as operating gains and losses after the determination of net income from providing services

Figure A2. Typical Income Statement

Medical Center
Statement of Revenues and Expenses
for the Years Ended June 30, 19x2 and 19x1

	19x2	19x1
Operating Revenues:		
Net patient service revenue	42,547,228	40,075,756
Other operating revenue	1,131,716	1,085,983
Total operating revenues	43,678,944	41,161,739
Operating Expenses:		
Salaries and wages	18,417,626	16,742,397
Payroll taxes and benefits	3,422,329	2,992,994
Professional fees	2,161,173	1,811,640
Supplies and other expenses	12,546,593	12,456,113
Provision for bad debts	1,025,728	230,189
Depreciation and amortization	2,906,091	2,876,525
Interest expense	1,520,809	1,758,331
Total Operating Expenses	42,000,281	38,868,189
Income from Operations	1,678,663	2,293,550
Nonoperating Gains (Losses)		
Investment income, net	693,487	567,292
Other expenses	---	(90,000)
Total Nonoperating Revenues	693,487	477,292
Excess of Revenues over Expenses	$ 2,372,150	$ 2,770,842

to patients. Interest earned from investments would not typically be shown as patient care revenues and should be shown after net patient care income has been determined in order to correctly identify the revenues earned from providing service to patients. in health maintenance organizations, interest earned can be shown as an operating revenue.

Expenses are typically presented on a functional basis and reflect the amounts expended to provide the services responsible for the revenues shown in the income statement.

Income statement accounts are considered to be temporary accounts, because they are zeroed out at the end of each accounting period to prepare them for the next accounting period.

The Statement of "Cash Flow"

The third financial statement that is required by GAAP is the statement of "cash flow." This statement uses data from the balance sheet and income statement to provide information on determining the factors accounting for changes in the cash balances of the organization resulting from the provision of services, investing decisions, and financing decisions for the period covered by the financial statements.

122

The statement of cash flow can be an important indicator of financial solvency. This statement separates the effects of normal operating activities from financing and investing activities. In other words, the effects of three major strategies and determinants of fiscal success are separated and shown in terms of their cash flow impact. A typical statement of cash flow is shown in figure A-3, page 124.

Financial Statement Analysis

An analysis of financial statements can be accomplished by several methods. Single point estimates can be obtained for comparison with other institutions, or external standards. A trend line is sometimes useful to identify possible problem areas. Both point and trend analysis are important for management information, but trend analysis has the added benefit of not requiring external comparison data. Because of the dissimilarity of many institutions, point comparisons can be very misleading. The accounts in the balance sheet and the income statements can be analyzed on a percentage basis. Common size and vertical analysis provides information on changes in the structure of the statements in terms of percentages. These composition ratios can indicate when profit margins are shrinking and what is causing the decrease—for example, when certain asset categories are increasing in relationship to the total asset structure. An analysis of two statements is generally more effective than single estimates.

Another commonly used analysis technique is computation and comparison of ratios. Ratios can be grouped into specific management areas to aid in analysis. Four key management areas are:

✦ Liquidity—Can the organization meet its current obligations?

✦ Turnover—Are the organization's assets being used effectively?

✦ Performance—Are the organization's assets being used efficiently?

✦ Capitalization—How are the assets being financed?

A summary of the ratios is included in figure A-4, page 125.

Sample Analysis of the Financial Statements

Using the data from figures A-1, A-2, and A-3 and the ratios from figure A-4, the following analysis could be accomplished for the sample provider:

Liquidity Ratios

Current Ratio = $\dfrac{11,375,301}{7,632,589}$ = 1.49

Figure A3. Statements of Cash Flow

Medical Center
Statements of Cash Flow
for the Years Ended June 30, 19x2 and 19x1

	19x2	19x1
Cash Flows from Operating Activities:		
Excess of revenues over expenses	$ 2,372,150	$ 2,770,842
Adjustments to excess of revenues over expenses		
Depreciation and amortization	2,906,091	2,867,525
Bad Debt Expense	1,025,720	230,189
Less contractual allowances and actual write-offs	(11,398,368)	(8,672,864)
(Gain) Loss on sale of property, plant, and equipment	36,162	(19,346)
Restricted donations and grants	210,180	11,929
Expenditure of restricted donations and grants	31,622	(57,345)
Changes in operating assets and liabilities		
(Increase) decrease in:		
Accounts receivable	(1,900,617)	(1,808,847)
Other accounts receivable	77,159	33,131
Reimbursement settlement receivable	8,067	7,318
Inventory of supplies	17,103	(90,284)
Prepaid expenses	27,463	126,828
Deferred professional liability costs	164,000	(164,000)
Accounts payable	372,913	(303,320)
Accrued payroll, payroll taxes, and employee benefits	99,689	(33,391)
Accrued interest payable	(40,895)	(3,466)
Other current liabilities	(94,775)	(28,864)
Reimbursement settlement payable	144,062	521,561
Other liabilities & deferred revenues	(83,680)	162,320
Net cash provided by operating activities	**$5,309,170**	**$4,222,780**

	19x2	19x1
Cash Flows from Investing Activities:		
Purchase of property, plant, and equipment	$(1,506,819)	$(2,814,626)
Proceeds from sale of property, plant, and equipment	112,741	29,499
Increase in assets whose use is limited	(2,244,553)	(337,626)
Net cash provided by investing activities	(3,638,631)	(3,122,753)
Cash Flows from Financing Activities:		
Principle payments on long-term debt	(2,404,400)	(1,285,400)
Increase in deferred financing costs		(17,550)
Net cash provided by financing activities	(2,404,400)	(1,302,950)
Net Decrease in Cash and Cash Equivalents	(733,861)	(202,923)
Cash and Cash Equivalents at Beginning of Year	1,125,628	1,328,551
Cash and Cash Equivalents at End of Year	$ 391,767	$ 1,125,628

Figure A4. Summary of Ratios

Liquidity

Current Ratio	=	$\dfrac{\text{Current Assets}}{\text{Current Liabilities}}$
Daily Cash Outflow	=	$\dfrac{\text{Operating Expenses—Noncash Expenses}}{\text{Days in Period}}$
Days of Cash Outflow Available	=	$\dfrac{\text{Cash}}{\text{Daily Cash Flow}}$
Times Interest Coverage	=	$\dfrac{\text{Revenues in Excess of Expenses from Operations+ Interest Expense}}{\text{Interest Expense}}$
Debt Service Ratio	=	$\dfrac{\text{Revenues in Excess of Expenses from Operations + Interest + Depreciation + Annual Debt Service Requirements}}{\text{Annual Debt Service}}$
Working Capital per Bed	=	$\dfrac{\text{Working Capital}}{\text{Available Beds}}$

Turnover Ratios

Asset Turnover	=	$\dfrac{\text{Net Operating Revenue}}{\text{Total Assets}}$
Accounts Receivable Turnover	=	$\dfrac{\text{Net Operating Revenue}}{\text{Net Accounts Receivable}}$
Inventory Turnover	=	$\dfrac{\text{Supply Expense}}{\text{Inventory}}$
Average Daily Patient Revenue	=	$\dfrac{\text{Net Operating Revenue}}{\text{Number of Days}}$
Average Collection Period	=	$\dfrac{\text{Net Accounts Receivable}}{\text{Average Daily Patient Revenue}}$
Average Daily Operating Expenses	=	$\dfrac{\text{Operating Expenses}}{\text{Number of Days}}$
Accounts Payable Payment Period	=	$\dfrac{\text{Accounts Payable}}{\text{Number of Days}}$

Performance Ratios

Operating Margin	=	$\dfrac{\text{Revenues in Excess of Expenses from Operations}}{\text{Net Revenues}}$
Return on Assets	=	$\dfrac{\text{Revenues in Excess of Expenses from Operations}}{\text{Total Assets}}$
Return on Fund Balance	=	$\dfrac{\text{Revenues in Excess of Expenses from Operations}}{\text{Fund Balance}}$
Pre-Financing Return on Assets	=	$\dfrac{\text{Revenues in Excess of Expenses from Operations+ Interest}}{\text{Total Assets}}$
Pre-Financing Return on Fund Balance and Long Term Debt	=	$\dfrac{\text{Revenues in Excess of Expenses from Operations+ Interest}}{\text{Fund Balance + Long-Term Debt}}$

Capitalization Ratios

Total Debt to Fund Balance	=	$\dfrac{\text{Total Debt}}{\text{Fund Balance}}$
Long-Term Debt to Total Assets	=	$\dfrac{\text{Long-Term Debt}}{\text{Total Assets}}$
Total Debt to Total Capitalization	=	$\dfrac{\text{Total Debt}}{\text{Total Assets}}$

$$\begin{array}{lll}
\text{Daily Cash} \\
\text{Outflow}
\end{array} = \dfrac{42,000,281 - (2,906,091 + 1,025,720)}{365} = \$104,297$$

$$\begin{array}{lll}
\text{Days of Cash} \\
\text{Outflow} \\
\text{Available}
\end{array} = \dfrac{391,767}{104,297} = 3.76 \text{ days}$$

$$\begin{array}{lll}
\text{Times} \\
\text{Interest} \\
\text{Covered}
\end{array} = \dfrac{2,372,150 + 1,520,809}{1,520,809} = 2.56 \text{ times}$$

Analysis: The provider has a satisfactory current ratio, but the days of cash outflow are minimal—collection of accounts receivable or short-term loans will be necessary to meet operating expenses.

Turnover Ratios

$$\begin{array}{lll}
\text{Asset} \\
\text{Turnover}
\end{array} = \dfrac{43,678,944}{42,130,623} = 1.04 \text{ times/year}$$

$$\begin{array}{lll}
\text{Accounts} \\
\text{Receivable} \\
\text{Turnover}
\end{array} = \dfrac{43,678,944}{8,399,210} = 5.2 \text{ times/year}$$

$$\begin{array}{lll}
\text{Inventory} \\
\text{Turnover}
\end{array} = \dfrac{12,546,593}{356,798} = 35.16 \text{ days}$$

$$\begin{array}{lll}
\text{Average} \\
\text{Daily} \\
\text{Revenue}
\end{array} = \dfrac{43,678,944}{365} = \$119,668$$

$$\begin{array}{lll}
\text{Average} \\
\text{Collection} \\
\text{Period}
\end{array} = \dfrac{8,399,210}{119,668} = 70.19 \text{ days}$$

$$\begin{array}{lll}
\text{Average} \\
\text{Daily} \\
\text{Supply Expense}
\end{array} = \dfrac{12,546,593}{365} = \$34,374$$

$$\begin{array}{lll}
\text{Accounts} \\
\text{Payable} \\
\text{Payment Period}
\end{array} = \dfrac{2,326,387}{34,374} = 67.68 \text{ days}$$

Analysis: Utilization of assets is average, as measured by the asset turnover of 1.04. The accounts receivable collection period of 70 days indicates some follow-up in this area would be useful, while the accounts payable cycle of 67.68 days means that bills are not paid promptly.

Performance Ratios

Operating Margin $= \dfrac{2,372,150}{43,678,944} = .054$

Return on Assets $= \dfrac{2,372,150}{42,130,623} = .0563$

Return on Fund Balance $= \dfrac{2,372,150}{22,019,974} = .1077$

Prefinancing Return on Assets $= \dfrac{2,372,150 + 1,520,809}{42,130,623} = .092$

Analysis: The owner has a reasonable operating margin (.054). The return on fund balance is high (10.77 percent) because of use of short-term credit in current liabilities.

Capitalization Ratios

Total Debt to Fund Balances $= \dfrac{42,130,623 - 22,019,974}{22,019,974} = \dfrac{20,110,649}{22,019,974} = .91$

Long-Term Debt to Total Assets $= \dfrac{12,325,500}{42,130,623} = .29$

Total Debt to Total Assets $= \dfrac{42,130,623 - 22,019,974}{42,130,623} = \dfrac{20,110,649}{42,130,623} = .48$

Analysis: The provider has 50 percent of capital from debt sources, which, in most cases, would be considered high. This may or may not be a problem, depending on the certainty of the payment process. If accounts receivable are sound, there should be no problem in paying off the debt. It might be prudent to add more long-term capital, either through retained earnings or a fund drive from the community.

Appendix B. Basic Budgeting Techniques

Types of Budgets

Budget preparation requires management to make certain assumptions about past expenditures. The first approach, known as an incremental approach, assumes that last year's expenses were correct and that these figures need to be adjusted only for changes in policies, technology, or volume. Incremental budgeting is one of the more commonly used techniques, but it does not give solid indications of where savings can be made or when more efficient management would reduce costs.

Program budgeting focuses on the major activities to be performed instead of on the organizational units. For example, possible programs would include dietary, housekeeping, nursing, maintenance, pharmacy, social service activities, laundry, security, medical clinics, occupational therapy, etc. Costs and revenues are developed for each program and in turn are allocated to the various departments responsible for providing the service. Major problems occur in this type of budget preparation when the programs become the responsibility of more than one supervisor. It is difficult to control expenditures when more than one person is responsible, and the allocation process is never completely objective. This is one of the major weaknesses of program budgeting; however, it can be selectively applied to a one-department program such as laboratory or imaging. A sample program budget format for a hospital dietary department is shown in Figure B1, right.

A different approach, zero-base budgeting, involves determination of inputs and outputs for various activities in the organization. For example, each departmental unit is broken down into discrete activities called

---

Figure B1. Sample Program Budget

Program: Dietary

Purpose: To provide nutritional food service with an appetizing appearance in accordance with approved dietary requirements.

Resources: (Based on 85% Occupancy)

	Fixed	Variable
Dietitian	x	
Cooks	x	
Helpers	x	
Food Costs		x
Supplies		x
Equipment	x	
Space	x	
Utilities	x	

Total Program Costs

Budget Equation:
Total Fixed Costs + Total Variable Costs = Total Program Costs;
Total Variable Costs = Total Meals Served times Variable Cost of Meals

---

128

decision packages. These decision packages are funded at specified levels and an output is determined for each funding level. In a sense, the activities must be justified from zero. The administrator and supervisors review each decision package and, through a ranking process, determine what level of funding to approve. An example of the decision package is shown in figures B2 and B3, pages 130 and 131.

Zero-base budgeting can be time-consuming and requires active participation by all supervisors. Accomplished properly, it provides a wealth of information about the activities of the organization. Incremental budgeting is the other extreme, because the amount that was approved last year becomes the starting amount for the new budget period. Program budgeting lies somewhere between the two extremes and has neither the maximum benefits of zero-base budgeting nor the lower cost of the incremental approach.

Flexible and Static Budgeting

Identification of variable and fixed cost components of cost categories makes it possible to use flexible budgeting techniques. A flexible budget is a budget that is adjusted for volume changes. For example, if nurse staffing is based on patient days, the budget allowance for nurse staffing would change with changes in patient activity level. Nursing administration costs, in comparison, are relatively fixed for reasonable ranges of patient activity.

Suppose 65,700 patient days were budgeted for a hospital's revenue projections. If we required 2.5 RN hours per patient day, then our budgeted RN hours would be 65,700 x 2.5 = 164,250. These hours could then be converted to a dollar cost by extending them at the average RN hourly rate. If that were $12 per hour, the total budgeted cost would be $1,971,000. If we did not adjust this budgeted amount for variation in patient days, we would be using a static budget approach.

A static budget approach to making judgments about organizational performance would take the planned budget as the basis against which to compare actual RN salary costs during the period. This adherence to a planned budgeted amount when the costs are variable can lead to dysfunctional managerial decisions. For example, if patient days turn out to be less than planned, the budget for RN salaries would be too loose, and even if actual RN costs were equal or slightly less than the budgeted amount, RNs would not have been used efficiently. If patient days turn out to be greater than planned, strict adherence to the budgeted RN costs would result in fewer RN hours being available for each patient day, and a reduction in the quality of care could result.

Flexible budgeting adjusts the planned budget for changes in levels of activity. For example, assume actual nursing costs were $1,971,000. Under the static budget concept, the variance would be zero. But if we also assume that the number of patient days was only 64,000, compared to the 65,700 that were planned, a flexible budgeting approach would tell us that the variance is not zero: A total of 64,000 patient days would require only 160,000 (64,000 x 2.5) RN hours compared

---

Figure B2. Decision Packages

Sample Format

1. Level of funding for this activity.
   Minimum level: amount of funding required without which this activity cannot be performed.[*]
   Same dollars: amount of funding equal to last year's budget.
   Same effort: amount of funding required to perform same level of activity as in last budget period.
   Maximum level: activities that would be performed if funding were increased over last year.[*]

2. Activity name and any identifying number used. For example, medical records admitting #MR-1.

3. Name of cost center where activity is performed. For example, medical records.

4. Date of preparation.

5. Number of pages in package.

6. Name of preparer of decision package.

7. Approval authority for this cost center.

8. Brief description of activity. For example, this activity consists of accessing the patient into the health care system. Admitting documents and appropriate health care personnel assigned.

9. The resources required for this package would be determined for specific categories. Last year's budgeted amount would be compared with this package, and the percentage change noted.

10. Activity measurements are typically divided into effectiveness and efficiency. Effectiveness measures include meeting JACHO objectives for this activity. For example, for the medical records admitting activity, this might include such factors as: (1) all patients desiring admission will be seen promptly and accurately; (2) proper health care personnel will be notified on a timely basis; (3) medical records will be prepared and maintained; (4) proper collection procedures will be instituted. Efficiency measures would concentrate on establishing more specific measure factors, such as (1) no patient will wait more than 10 minutes to be admitted; (2) the patient will be moved to his or her assigned room within 20 minutes; (3) medical records will be prepared with no more than 5 percent errors; (4) collections forms and procedures will be implemented no later than two hours after admission.

11. This section should stress the benefits to be realized from approving this package. For example, this level of activity will enable the organization to meet accreditation standards or provide minimum levels of information in the medical records.

12. This section should stress the impact of not funding this level of activity. For example, the medical records function will not meet accreditation and/or legal requirements.

13. This section would list other packages developed for this activity and their ranking by the preparer.

14. This section would include data on how other reviewers ranked this package in relation to all other packages being reviewed.

---

[*] The minimum and maximum levels of funding should be established by top management during the planning period. For example, the minimum level might be established as 80 percent of last year's budget amount, with the maximum set at 120 percent.

Figure B2. Decision Packages (continued)

Sample Package

1. (Minimum Level)_____ (Same Dollars) _____ (Same Effort)_____ (Maximum Level) _____
2. Activity Name and Number_____ 3. Responsibility Unit _____
4. Date_____ 5. Page _____ of_____
6. Prepared by _____ 7. Approved by _____
8. Description of Activity: _____
9. Resources Required (this package):

	Current Year	Proposed Budget	% Change
Personnel (FTE)			
Salaries			
Fringe			
Equipment			
Supplies			
Other			
Totals			

10. Measures of Performance:

Effectiveness_____

Efficiency _____

11. Benefits of Approval:
12. Impact of Not Funding:
13. Other Decision Packages for This Activity (attach details):

Same Dollar	Ranking_____
Same Effort	Ranking_____
120%	Ranking_____

14. Ranking of This Decision Package

By Preparing Management Level	Number_____ of _____	Packages
By First Reviewing Management Level	Number_____ of _____	Packages
By Second Reviewing Management Level	Number_____ of _____	Packages

---

Figure B3. Decision Package Ranking Form

Organizational Level _____ Number of Packages _____

Date _____ Page_____ of_____

Prepared by_____ Next Reviewing Level_____

Priority Number	Package Name	Decision Unit	Type Package	Amount of Funding	Cumulative Funding	FTE	Comments
1	Medical Records	Administration	80%	$50,000	$50,000	5	Medicaid Requirement
2	Linen Change	Housekeeping	80%	$30,000	$80,000	2	Accreditation Requirement

to the 164,250 RN hours that were planned. The budget for 160,000 RN hours should be $1,920,000, (160,000 x $12), producing an unfavorable variance of $51,000 ($1,920,000 - $1,971,000).

In most organizations, the flexible budget approach offers a more realistic assessment of performance and a better approach to cost control. For many providers where most of the costs are relatively fixed, the static budget approach may be adequate. But if variable costs, even if relatively small, can be determined, the flexible approach provides more detailed information and can identify excess as well as insufficient resource utilization.

Appendix C. Standard Costs and Variance Analysis

Standard Costs

The development of standard costs requires input from all relevant decision-makers. For example, in larger providers, the supervisor, the purchasing agent, the human resources officer, and other key personnel should be included, because every standard consists of both an estimated cost per resource unit and an estimate of the number of units of resource to be used. For example, the nursing supervisor would be responsible for determining the number of RN hours required to provide high-quality care. The human resources officer may be responsible for establishing competitive salaries. For supplies, the purchasing agent could develop the estimated costs per item, while the central supply supervisor could control the usage rate. By determining the cost and usage standards in advance, the performance reports become more meaningful for control purposes. A sample computation is shown in Figure C1, page 135.

Standard costs can also be useful in simplifying the accounting system. For example, items in supply would be carried at the standard costs, not the actual amounts paid. Given a standard of raw food cost per patient day, the number of estimated patient days times that standard cost per day would give the total budgeted raw food cost for the period under study. Variances would be handled through the preparation of the financial statements at the end of the operating period. The same system could be used for salaries and wages. In addition, the development of standard costs makes it easier to establish a rate for a new service based on cost.

A standard cost system can be a vital part of the budgeting and control process. Managers intuitively establish standards on the basis of their experiences as to what something should cost. A formalized system makes the benefits of this experience available to all the employees.

Variance Analysis

If proper standards have been developed before the fact, the actual results can be compared to those standards and corrective action can be taken when appropriate. For example, consider the following situation for a laboratory test:

Test A—
Technician standard hours: 3.5 per test
Technician standard cost per hour: $12.00
Estimated number of tests for the month: 480

Budget allowance:
   480 x 3.5 hours = 1,680 hours; 1,680 x $12.00 = $20,160 Total Cost
Actual technician hours used = 1,740
Actual salary expenses = $21,500
Actual tests performed = 520

The variances could be computed in this manner:

Total variance = $21,500 - $20,160 = $1,340 (unfavorable)

This $1,340 unfavorable variance can be further explained as follows:

Wage Variance

Actual wages paid	$21,500
Actual hours x standard wage (1,740 hrs x $12.00)	-20,880
Wage variance	620 (unfavorable)

Efficiency Variance

Standard hours for actual tests (520 x 3.5 hrs)	1,820
Actual hours used	-1,740
	80 hours (favorable)

At $12.00/hour, the value of these extra hours is $960.

Volume Variance

Actual volume of tests	520
Planned volume of tests	-480
Test volume variance	40 (unfavorable from a cost perspective)

40 tests x 3.5 hours x $12.00 = $1,680 (unfavorable) or

Planned budget at 520 tests	$21,840
Planned budget at 480 tests	-20,160
	$ 1,680 (unfavorable)

Net Variance

Volume Variance	$1,680 (unfavorable)
Wage Variance	620 (unfavorable)
Efficiency Variance	-960 (favorable)
	$1,340 (unfavorable)

134

Figure C1. Computation of Standard Cost per Lab Procedure

Station 3

Variable Costs (based on required hours x salary rates)	Per Day
Supervisor wages	$ 2.35
Technician wages	1.59
Clerical wages	4.29
Supplies	.44
Total Variable Costs	**$ 8.67**

Direct Fixed Costs (based on total budget/lab tests)	
Contract Service	$ .85
Consulting	.50
Rentals	.03
Total Direct Fixed Costs	**1.38**

Total Direct Costs per Test	**$10.05**

Indirect Expenses (based on total budget/lab tests)	
Housekeeping	$ 1.17
Laundry	1.16
Security	.73
Maintenance	2.96
Property Taxes, Insurance, Depreciation	3.47
Administrative	5.55
Total Allocated Cost per test	**$15.04**

Total Cost per Test	$25.09
Desired Profit Percentage (10%)	2.51
Average Rate per Test	$27.60

Appendix D. Cost/Volume/Profit Models

Based on our understanding of cost behavior, a tool can be developed that will enable managers to make better forecasts of volume and better estimates of what the corresponding rate should be, or to assess more accurately the effects of changes in variable or fixed costs. To review our understanding of cost behavior, the following definitions are presented:

✦ Variable costs are assumed to vary directly in proportion to the volume of services provided.

✦ Fixed costs are assumed not to vary with volume changes.

Given these two basic assumptions, the cost structure for the service can be expressed as follows:

(1) Total Costs (TC) = Total Fixed Costs (TFC) + Total Variable Costs (TVC); TC = TFC + TVC.

(2) TVC = Variable Costs per Unit of Service (VCU) x Volume (or number of units) of service (Q). Therefore, equation (1) can also be expressed as TC = TFC + (VCU x Q).

(3) Average Total Cost (ATC) = Total Cost per unit of volume or service = $\frac{TC}{Q}$

$$\frac{TC}{Q} = \frac{TFC}{Q} + \frac{TVC}{Q}$$

$$\frac{TFC}{Q} = AFC$$

$$\frac{TVC}{Q} = \frac{(VCU)\,(Q)}{Q} = VCU = AVC$$

$$ATC = AFC + AVC = \frac{TFC}{Q} + VCU$$

The first three equations can be expressed in the following model when revenues and profits requirements are introduced.

(4) Total Revenues (TR)[1] = Rate per Unit of Service (R) x Volume of service (Q); TR = R x Q.

Desired Profit or Income (I) can be expressed as a dollar requirement or as a percentage of total revenue requirement and on a before- or after-tax basis.[2]

---

[1] Total revenues are defined as the amount expected to be collected from all patients.

[2] This works as well for nonprofit organizations. With a tax rate of zero, the before-tax and after-tax requirements are simply equal.

(5a) After-tax dollar requirement = I

Before-tax dollar requirement $= \dfrac{I}{(1 - \text{tax rate})}$

(5b) After-tax percentage of total revenue requirement = %TR

Before-tax percentage of total revenue requirement $= \dfrac{\%TR}{(1 - \text{tax rate})}$

The summary and complete model can be expressed as:

(6a) TR = TC + I **or**

$R \times Q = TFC + (VCU)(Q) + \dfrac{I}{(1 - \text{tax rate})}$

or, solving for R,

(7) $R = \dfrac{TFC}{Q} + VCU + \dfrac{I}{(1 - \text{tax rate}) \times Q}$

An example of how this can be used is to determine the rate that must be charged to obtain a desired level of profit.

Given:

TFC	=	$50,000
VCU	=	$11
Desired I (after taxes)	=	$10,000
Tax rate	=	37.5%
Q	=	5,000

Substituting:

$R = \dfrac{\$50,000}{5,000} + \$11 + \dfrac{\$10,000}{(1 - .375) * 5,000}$

$R = \$10 + \$11 + \dfrac{\$2}{(1 - .375) * 5,000} = \$10 + \$11 + \$3.20 = \$24.20$

This answer can be verified by completing a simplified income statement.

Total Revenue	5,000	x	$24.20	=	$121,000
Variable Costs	5,000	x	$11.00	=	$ 55,000
Contribution Margin	5,000	x	$13.20	=	$ 66,000

Total Fixed Costs	$ 50,000
Income Before Taxes	$ 16,000
Taxes at a 37 ½% Rate	$ 6,000
Income After Taxes	$ 10,000

The basic cost/volume/profit model of equation (7) can also be used, for example, to compare the effects of buying more equipment (increased fixed costs) with switching to outside suppliers on a fee-for-service basis (increased variable costs). Of course, the estimates going into the model do not have to be, indeed cannot be, precise. Few events in the future can be determined precisely. What is needed is an estimate of the reasonableness of the numbers. Is this rate reasonable? Can this quantity realistically be obtained? How sensitive are the results to alternative assumptions? The model allows the input necessary for this type of analysis.

Multiple Payers

For many departments, there is no single rate for services provided because of the varying amounts paid by different third-party payers. Each individual rate may reflect third-party regulations, competitive pressures, and/or managerial judgments about future costs, market dynamics, inflation, etc. Once individual rates have been estimated, the same approach described above can be used, but the single rate used in the model above becomes a weighted average of the various payer rates. In the example above, a single rate of $24.20 resulted. But this $24.20 could represent an average rate developed in the following manner:

	Proportion of Total Volume	x	Rate		
Medicare	30%	x	$20.00	=	$ 6.00
Medicaid	50%	x	15.40	=	$ 7.70
Charge-Based	20%	x	52.50	=	$10.50
	100%				
			Average Revenue		**$24.20**

The following example shows how the rate for a charge-based payer can be determined where multiple payers exist.

Given:

✦ 40,000 lab tests are forecast.
✦ The Medicare rate is $32.00 and Medicare is 40% of all activity .
✦ The Medicaid rate is $20.00 and Medicaid is 50% of all activity.
✦ Charge-based activity is 10% of all activity.
✦ Fixed costs are $600,000.
✦ Variable costs are $10.00 per lab test.
✦ The desired profit margin is $100,000 after taxes.
✦ The tax rate is 37½%.

What rate must be charged to charge-based payers to meet the desired profit margin? Using the model developed above and substituting the new information, the average rate would be:

$$R_A = [TFC + (VCU \times Q) + \frac{I}{(1 - \text{tax rate})}] \div Q$$

$$R_A = [\$600{,}000 + (\$10 \times 40{,}000) + \frac{\$100{,}000}{(1-.375)}] \div 40{,}000$$

$$R_A = \frac{\$600{,}000}{40{,}000} + \$10 + \frac{\$160{,}000}{40{,}000} = \$15 + \$10 + \$4 = \underline{\$29}$$

Using the weighted average approach developed above, the charge for charge-based payers would be:

	Proportion of Total Volume	x	Rate		
Medicare	40%	x	$32.00	=	$10.00
Medicaid	50%	x	20.00	=	$12.80
Charge-Based	10%	x	R_{Chg}	=	$?
	100%				
			Average Revenue		**$29.00**

R_{Chg} = ($29.00 - $10.00 - $12.80) divided by .10 = $6.20 ÷ .10 = $62.00, the required charge for charge-based payers.

These results can be verified using the income statement approach:

Revenues

Medicare	40%	x	40,000	x	$32.00	=	$ 512,000
Medicaid	50%	x	40,000	x	22.00	=	400,000
Charge-Based	10%	x	40,000	x	62.00	=	248,000
			Total Revenue			=	**$1,160,000**

Expenses

Fixed Costs	$600,000
Variable Costs (40,000 x $10)	$400,000
Total Costs =	$1,000,000
Profit before taxes	$ 160,000
Taxes at 37½%	60,000
Profit after taxes	$ 100,000

If the mix of the various payers changes, the effect on the rate can also be determined and adjustments can be made accordingly.

A Contribution Model

A short-cut approach to the cost/volume/profit model is one that focuses on the Contribution Margin (CM), or the difference between the Rate (R) and the Variable Cost per Unit (VCU). Through concentration on the contribution margin, answers can rapidly be obtained to the questions posed above. For example, the basic contribution model can be expressed as:

(8) $\text{TFC} + \dfrac{I}{1 - \text{tax rate}} = Q \times CM$

where I is the desired after-tax income and CM is defined as (R - VCU). Given the numbers in the first example above:

R	=	$24.50
TFC	=	$50,000
VCU	=	$11
I	=	10,000
Tax rate	=	37½%
Q	=	Unknown

Substituting in the Equation (8):

$$\$50,000 + \dfrac{\$10,000}{1 - .375} = Q \times \$13.20$$

$$Q = \dfrac{\$50,000 + \$16,000}{\$13.20}$$

$$= \dfrac{\$66,000}{\$13.20}$$

$$= 5,000$$

The contribution margin approach can also be used effectively to monitor and report on departmental activities. The basic format changes to define margin as the difference between total revenues and direct costs (TR - DC). Direct costs include all costs for which the department supervisor is responsible. For example, the department supervisor is responsible for salaries paid and supplies used. The depreciation on equipment used only in the department, any special maintenance, etc., are considered direct costs. Other costs, such as general administration, utilities, and housekeeping, are considered indirect costs, because they are not under the control of the department supervisor but are generally allocated. An example performance report might be:

Total Revenues	$100,000
Total Direct Costs	70,000
Direct Margin	$ 30,000
Allocated Indirect Costs	25,000
Departmental Income	$ 5,000

The direct margin should be the point of emphasis for the control process. The amount of indirect costs can be changed by the choice of allocation methods as well as by third-party payment regulations. Although the bottom line is a proper concern of senior managers, it is questionable whether it should be used to evaluate lower levels of supervisors, whose range of choice and control is limited.

Appendix E. Net Present Value Calculations

Assume that a proposal to be evaluated requires an initial cash investment of $1,000 and is expected to provide incremental cash inflows of $372 at the end of the first year and $1,296 at the end of the second year. The organization's overall WACC is estimated to be 20 percent during both years. This 20 percent rate means that the $1,000 investment should provide a total return of at least $1,200 if the proposed activity lasts just one year. But this proposal covers two years, and, while it provides only $372 in the first year, it also generates $1,296 in the second year. This means that we must evaluate both of the cash inflows to see if their combined value provides a total return sufficient to meet our 20 percent WACC.

To value flows over two years, we simply do what we already know how to do, but we do it twice:

	Incremental Operational Cash Flows	
Present Value at 20%	End of Year 1	End of Year 2

```
$ 900 ◄──── 2nd year flow ÷ by 1.20 twice ◄──────── $1,296
$ 310 ◄──── 1st year flow ÷ by 1.20 ◄──── $ 372           │
                                          +1,080   ÷  1.20
$1,210 ◄──── ÷ 1.20 ◄──────────────────── $1,452
```

Value of both inflows as of today	Value of both inflows as of the end of Year 1

-1,000 Value of initial outflow

$ 210 Net Present Value

Because the present value of the $1,000 initial cash outflow today is $1,000, the NPV of this proposal is $210. Obviously, this proposal is very desirable from a fiscal viewpoint.

A different way of arriving at the same result is as follows:

1. $1,000 invested at 20 percent for two years yields $1,440 = ($1,000 x 1.20 x 1.20). Therefore, if a proposal returned exactly $1,440 on a $1,000 investment after two years it would exactly meet the organization's WACC and have a net present value of zero.

2. But this proposal returns $372 after one year and $1,296 the second year. Because they're not the "same" kind of dollars, you can't just add $372 and $1,296. But you can adjust the $372 by *presuming* you could invest it at the same 20 percent rate that was applied above:

$372 x 1.20 = $ 446.40 (Value of first year payment at end of second year)
                1,296.00 Second year payment
        $1,742.40 Total return at end of second year

3. By comparing the $1,742 total return after two years to the $1,440 "breakeven" return from Step 1, you see that the proposal generates an extra $302.40 over "cost." This might well be called the "net *future* value" of the proposal, because the money shows up two years from now.

4. To convert net future value to net present value, you have to discount it back for two years. As discussed previously, you simply divide the $302.40 by the discount factor (in this case 1.20) twice, because two years of adjustment have to be made: $302.40 ÷ 1.20 = $252.00; $252.00 ÷ 1.20 = $210.00 = the net present value.

CHAPTER 10

Planning and Marketing: An External Perspective to Competitive Strategy

by Eric N. Berkowitz, PhD

Since the mid-1970s, the management of health care organizations has gone through a period of rapid change in response to an increasingly complex environment. One aspect of this change has been the introduction of marketing as a functional area within the management setting. Common to many traditional industries, marketing was considered a novel approach to respond to the increasing competitive environment being felt by many provider organizations in the mid-1970s. The purpose of this chapter is to discuss the meaning of marketing and how it affects on the planning process of organizations, as well as the key components to marketing strategy formulation.

The Nature of Marketing

Marketing is both a process and a philosophy. In integrating marketing into an organization, the hospital or the medical group must view the service offering not from the perspective of the provider, but rather from that of the buyer. To be market-driven is to be customer-responsive. In its simplest form, marketing may be defined as the process by which customer needs are identified and a product (or service) is developed in response to that need.[1] The service is delivered, priced, and promoted according to the best way to attract the consumer. In this perspective of marketing, there are four components of strategy that will be discussed in greater depth in this chapter. These four components, referred to as the four P's of marketing, or the marketing mix, are product, price, place, and promotion. All organizations have these four components in their control to some extent. That is, what products or services should be offered and at what price? How should these services be delivered or made accessible (place), and in what manner can the market be informed of the service's existence (promotion)?

Later in this chapter, each of these components is discussed in greater depth.

In considering a marketing approach in health care, the consumer is at the center of the process. It is the consumer's needs to which the organization responds. For most health care organizations, this definition of the consumer varies and rarely consists of a single constituency. Figure 1, below, shows some of the multiple markets that exist for a hospital, a multispecialty group practice, or a single program such as adolescent chemical dependency. The challenge for health care organizations in developing an effective marketing approach is balancing the often varying needs of each respective market with the clinical service quality issues of the provider.

Figure 1. Multiple Markets/Multiple Provider

Provider	Markets
Hospital	Patients Physicians Corporations HMOs
Multispecialty Group	Patients Physicians Corporations
Adolescent Chemical Dependency Program	Parents Judges Social Workers Third-Party Payers

The Market-Driven Planning Sequence

Recognizing that marketing is driven by the consumer has a significant implication for the planning process of the organization. Historically, health care organizations were not market-driven. Rather, planning occurred from an internal perspective. In the typical planning mode, the hospital or group might examine statistics on the market in terms of age or income, along with various epidemiological data of the primary and secondary service area. The confluence of these factors might lead to a decision that a particular service was or wasn't needed in the community. After committing to the development of the service, it was then left to the administrator or chief financial officer to determine the pricing for the service. No formal strategy was developed for the service beyond the offering of this new program. Scheduling, location of the satellite facility, or determining how the market would be informed of the service was left to the discretion of the providers of the service.

In a market-driven approach, the introduction of a new service occurs as the result of a very different set of activities. Often, providers within a group or hospital might suggest a new service, such as rehabilitation medicine or a scoliosis clinic. Prior to rolling out the service, an assessment of the market is made. Is there a demand for this new service? Are there other providers in the market? What price are buyers willing to pay for this offering? Where would users like to receive this service and during what hours? In a market-driven sequence, the definition of a service is really provided by the likely buyer or user of the service. The provider's role is to ensure clinical quality and to deliver the offering.

In considering the conditions that have existed for most health care organizations up to the mid-1970s, it is easy to understand why a market-based approach was never integrated into typical health care planning. For most of the 1950s, 1960s, and even 1970s, most communities were still underserved with regard to a range of clinical services or providers. In fact, for most hospitals and other medical institutions, this period was not one of great cost or utilization pressure. When a service was offered, the primary problem was typically that of trying to meet demand rather than to stimulate it. In the rare instance when a medical organization offered a new service that was not successful, it was often viewed by the board of trustees or physicians as a good learning experience. Why is a marketing-based approach now a more common occurrence? Rarely is the problem now facing medical organizations one of meeting demand. It is more likely a situation of trying to generate utilization or volume. Additionally, 15 or 20 years ago, most health care organizations were in relatively strong financial positions. A new clinical service that was not successful financially could be seen as a learning experience. Today, there are few health care organizations that can afford very many learning experiences.

It Begins with Research

Essential to effective marketing is the need to conduct marketing research.[2] As discussed previously, marketing involves an external to internal planning perspective. It is marketing research that provides this external perspective. It is not the purpose of this chapter to describe all the intricacies of marketing research methodologies. However, it is important to recognize that it is the rare successful marketing company that does not conduct marketing research on an ongoing basis.

Secondary data. Marketing research can be obtained from either primary or secondary data. Secondary data are data that were collected for purposes beyond the specific problem at hand. In health care, there are several commercial, secondary data sources that are often used consisting of:

✦ Census data—Companies such as Urban Decision Systems offer simplified ways of using census data by zip code.

✦ Syndicated marketing research—These are research efforts to which a health

145

care organization can subscribe to receive regular updates on particular topics. The National Research Corporation (NRC) publishes its annual *Healthcare Market Guide*, an annual survey of 100,00 households in the top 100 markets in the United States. These data provide perceptual information regarding hospitals in a particular market as well as other breakdowns of interest. NRC is just one of several companies now entering the syndicated market research data field in health care.[3]

With any secondary data, it is important to recognize their major limitation—the data were not collected for the specific institution or issue of concern. In using secondary market research data, one must always be concerned with the quality of the study, the timeliness of the data, the relevance of the sample, and whether the classifications of the data are worthwhile.

Primary data. Because of the limitations of secondary data, most organizations will collect primary data for a project of importance. Figure 2, page 147 shows common methods used in collecting primary data and the respective trade-offs with each technique. Increasingly in health care, focus groups are seen as a valuable tool. In focus groups 10-12 individuals are led through a series of relatively open-ended questions by a trained moderator. While not providing empirical numbers, focus groups can often reveal issues and concerns that can be explored further in a mail or phone survey. Focus groups are increasingly used in two different steps in the marketing research process. Many organizations use them at the beginning of the research process to reveal issues, such as what are the possible reasons why a radiology group isn't getting referrals. Or, focus groups can be used at the end of the research process to help explain the results in a survey. For example, a focus group might be constructed to better understand why 75 percent of the people indicated they were somewhat dissatisfied with the service of the emergency department.

No doubt all readers of this book have been at the receiving end of phone, mail, and personal interviews, so no definitions of each approach are needed. However, a few comments about each methodology may be helpful. In conducting personal and telephone interviews, it is important to use trained interviewers. The potential for bias with an untrained interviewer can make the data collection highly suspect. Phone interviewers are also a very valuable way to collect information quickly.[4] Mail surveys are difficult to conduct because of the nonresponse bias. While there are many methods for improving the response rates for mail surveys, the ultimate question is always whether the person who responded is in any way different from the individual who did not respond. Except for the cost savings of mail surveys, there is little else to speak to their advantage beyond protection of the identity of the respondent.

Product: The Foundation of Strategy

The focus of marketing strategy revolves around the product or service. In marketing, a central concept to developing product or service strategy is the *product*

Figure 2. Alternative Research Methodologies[*]

Approach Criteria	Research Methodology			
	Personal Interview	Telephone Survey	Mail Survey	Focus Groups
Economy	Most expensive	Avoids interviewer travel, relatively expensive. Trained interviewers needed.	Potentially lower costs (if response rate sufficient)	Relatively expensive
Interviewer bias	High likelihood of bias. Trust. Appearance.	Less than personal interviewer. No face-to-face contact. Suspicion of phone call.	Interviewer bias eliminated. Anonymity provided.	Need trained moderator.
Flexibility	Most flexible Responses can be probed. Assistance can be provided in completing forms. Observations can be made.	Cannot make observations. Probing possible to a degree.	Least flexible	Very flexible.
Sampling and respondent cooperation	Most complete sample possible, with sufficient call back strategy.	Limited to people with telephone. No answers. Refusals are common.	Mailing list Nonresponse a major problem.	Need close selection.

[*] Reprinted from Hillestad, S., and Berkowitz, E. *Health Care Marketing Plans: From Strategy to Action.* Second Edition. Rockville, Md.: Aspen Press, 1991, p. 100.

life cycle. The product life cycle concept assumes that all products (or services) go through four distinct stages; introduction, growth, maturity, and decline. Figure 3, page 149, shows a generalized product life cycle curve. On the X-axis is time, and the Y-axis represents sales or gross revenues. In each stage, market conditions change, which requires a change in organizational strategy. At the introduction stage, sales rise slowly. At growth, significant increases in sales occur, which level off during maturity. Ultimately, revenue drops during decline.

Introduction. In the introduction stage, the new service enters the market. For example, the first HMO opens in the community. With regard to marketing strategy, there is one overriding objective in the introduction stage—generate awareness for the new service. At this stage, promotion becomes important. Either advertising announcing the new service or strong personal sales efforts, such as informational lectures by physicians or others, are required to inform potential users of the service.

147

In terms of pricing decisions, there are two typical options at the introduction stage—*skimming* or *penetration*. In rolling out a new product or service, there are some distinct advantages to a low or penetration pricing strategy. Typically, this approach makes acceptance of the new service easier, because the buyer's financial risk is reduced. Also, it has the effect of delaying competitors from entering the market. Any new competitor must attempt to price lower, which is often difficult with a real penetration pricing strategy. For many service businesses, however, this pricing approach is risky. When the estimation of demand for a new service is somewhat difficult to accurately gauge, a penetration pricing strategy may lead to some capacity problems in the organization. That is, as often happens for a medical service, demand can be greater than can be met through the staffing of the clinical service. While the organization is pleased at the market response, the delay in access to the new service can create ill will in the marketplace.

When capacity is an issue, it may be wise to price high (skimming). In this way, the buyers who truly value the service will purchase it. The provider can gradually meet a larger potential demand by lowering prices as facility capacity expands. Skimming also allows the organization to recoup its often high investment costs in setting up a new program before more aggressive price cutting occurs as other competitors enter the market. In a service business, such as health care, a high price also plays an important role in terms of image. That is, for many buyers there is often a perceived price/quality relationship that is enhanced by a higher price. The major disadvantage of a high price is that it encourages competition to enter the market. Other providers, seeing the high price being charged for a particular service, may feel that they could enter the market, offer a program of similar quality, and be more attractive to the market by undercutting the higher priced alternative. This type of market condition has been seen among HMOs that are competing in a particular city. As new competitors enter the market, they are accompanied by drastic cutting of premiums.

In the introduction stage of a new service, there is one other aspect that is essential from a marketing perspective. The product quality must meet customers' expectations. The quickest way to kill a new product is to offer it to the market before internal problems are worked out. For example, aggressive promoting of an industrial medicine program is essential in the introduction stage of the life cycle. Yet, if there are staffing problems or physical plant constraints or logistics that have not been worked out, a market disaster is sure to occur. Corporations are attracted by the promotion of the new industrial medicine program. Salespeople sign contracts. Workers begin to show up for physicals, rehabilitation, or treatment for job-related injuries, and the health care organization does not have the resources or capacity to meet the demand in a timely, efficient fashion. It is very unlikely that these dissatisfied buyers will be willing to sign contracts in the second year on the basis of assurances from the provider that the "kinks" have been worked out.

Growth. The second stage of the product life cycle is the period of the most rapid increases in sales. It is in this stage that competitors enter the market. At the

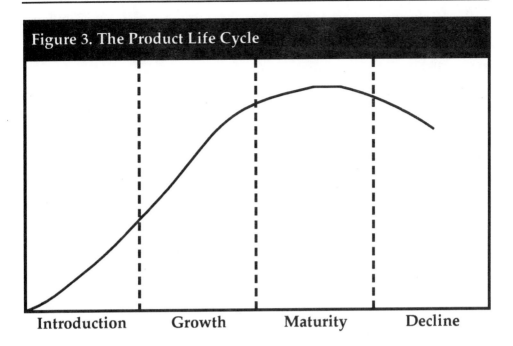

Figure 3. The Product Life Cycle

Introduction　　　Growth　　　Maturity　　　Decline

growth stage, the focus of attention becomes locking up the referral flow for patients. In the HMO market, for example, when new competitors entered the scene, the early HMOs tried to lock up existing providers with favorable terms conditional on the providers' signing exclusive contracts. For the new entrants at the growth stage, the key is to develop a differential advantage relative to the first provider. Typically, the source of the differential advantage is relative to some aspect of the marketing mix. The second or third medical group to enter might offer extended hours or more satellite locations, or the new HMO might require a lower premium.

Maturity. The third phase of the life cycle is when sales begin to level off. Often at this point, marginal competitors will begin to leave the market. In many communities, the HMO business is in this stage. In some parts of the country, plans have disappeared, and there is consolidation among the remaining plans. The focus of attention at this stage is to maintain market share. Because the market is mature, any lost customers will not be easily replaced. Customer retention is the key. Also at this point of the life cycle, it is important to look for new opportunities or service alternatives to get back up on the growth curve.

Decline. The final stage is the period of declining sales. Typically, at this stage the organization must make the decision to drop the product or determine another efficient way of providing the service. In the past few years in certain markets, some hospitals have dropped obstetrics or pediatrics. Other hospitals, in an attempt to offer a service, have signed agreements to have the service provided by a third party. This stage is often the most difficult for companies to manage. In traditional industries, it is often believed that a disproportionate amount of management time and attention is spent in dealing with declining products.

Price: The Key to Revenue

As previously discussed, price plays an important role for an organization in setting the strategy for the introduction of a new service. Yet it is important to recognize the difference between the marketing and the finance perspectives regarding price. In most health care settings, the issue of price is one that is decided internally. That is, what are the internal cost, the overhead allocation, and the margin? It is on these determinations that pricing decisions are made in conjunction with reimbursement constraints.

From a marketing perspective, these internal pricing concerns are important. But, in consideration of the external to internal perspective of marketing, it is the market's willingness to pay a determined price that guides strategy. That is, how much does the market want to pay for an industrial medicine program? Does the market want the package of services delivered at a bundled or unbundled price? How price sensitive is the buyer? The difference between marketing and finance with regard to price is the difference between the floor and the ceiling.

In an internal perspective, the administrator or chief financial officer is always concerned about cost and overhead. This is the floor. Pricing below this level leads to a loss. From a marketing perspective, the focus of concern is external, on the ceiling. How high would the market go for a particular service if it saw a value added to it? The difference between the ceiling and the floor represents the margin.

To a large extent, changes in the computer industry reflect the difficulty of premium pricing in health care. Ten years ago, as an emerging industry, computer companies, such as IBM, followed a premium pricing strategy. For a new product with a lot of risk for the buyer, the value added to an IBM computer was the brand name of the organization. IBM was the industry standard. Early buyers of computers can remember the term "IBM compatible" as the risk factor when one of these name brand alternatives wasn't purchased. In recent years, however, the products of the computer industry have become commodity goods. It is difficult to premium price a commodity product. IBM, along with manufacturers of other well-known brand names, has seen a precipitate decline in its margins, because consumers are no longer willing to pay a premium. The value added is gone.

In health care, the pricing challenge is the same. Ideally, an organization would always prefer to price high. A larger margin is more profitable and allows more room for error. As health care moves to more of a commodity position, however, obtaining a price differential from the buyer is increasingly difficult.

Place: Getting the Service

The third component of marketing strategy is often called place, or distribution. In the traditional product setting, it involves all the decisions of moving a product from producer to consumer. In developing marketing strategies around this component, the organization is concerned with where a service is to be offered, what hours it might be available, or how it will be accessed. In health care, place or distribution issues focus on decisions regarding the flow of patients through the system. Figure 4, below, shows several alternative patient flows through the system, called in marketing the *channel of distribution*. As can been in column A, the simplest flow of patients is to the primary care doctor. As one moves from B through D, other intermediaries often intervene, be they specialists, hospitals, tertiary hospitals, or HMO companies.

In terms of dealing with patient flow, the goal is to always control this channel of distribution. There are two common strategies often used in marketing, referred to as either *push* or *pull*. In a push strategy, the organization develops an approach to work through the intermediaries in the channel. For example, in channel C, the hospital wants to get patients from the physicians. Often, these intermediaries, the doctors, have privileges at more than one hospital. In developing a push strategy, the administrator wants to work through the doctors. One approach might consist of developing a medical office building and giving discounted rent to the doctors. In this way, the physician located next to a particular hospital might encourage patients to be admitted to that facility. Another approach, less cost intensive, might consist of programs to make doctors feel positively toward a particular facility. Weekend retreats, valet parking for physicians, and good lunches in the doctors' lounge are all relatively low cost ways of encouraging the intermediaries in the channel to direct patient flow. These are all push strategies that work through the intermediaries.

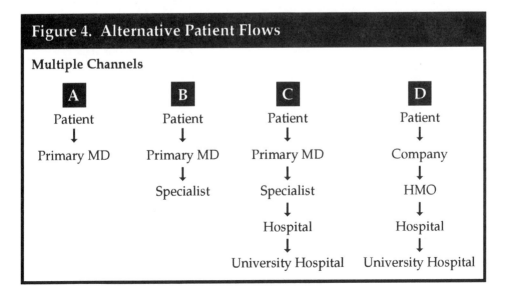

Figure 4. Alternative Patient Flows

Multiple Channels

A	B	C	D
Patient	Patient	Patient	Patient
↓	↓	↓	↓
Primary MD	Primary MD	Primary MD	Company
	↓	↓	↓
	Specialist	Specialist	HMO
		↓	↓
		Hospital	Hospital
		↓	↓
		University Hospital	University Hospital

The alternative to push approaches is pull strategies. In a pull strategy, the organization bypasses the intermediaries and goes directly to the user, in this case the patient. An HMO, for example, occasionally faces resistance when trying to have its plan offered in a particular company. If the company (figure 4, column D) does not offer the HMO, employees can never access the plan. In this case, the intermediary must be bypassed. The HMO might run an advertisement that says, "If your company does not offer the XYZ HMO, you can't pick one of the better plans available—Ask your boss why not?" The goal of such an approach is to encourage potential patients to approach the company and demand that the plan be offered. A similar pull strategy is being seen by many hospitals that advertise a particular "Center of Excellence." The purpose is to get the patient to ask the doctor about being admitted to that institution if the problem is relevant. Or, if the doctor does not have privileges at the facility, the patient can bypass the intermediary and go directly to the facility. In order for a pull strategy to work effectively, the organization or service must have very strong brand name recognition. Mayo, for example, can benefit from a pull strategy. A patient told of a major problem might say, "I'm not staying locally, I'm going to the Mayo Clinic." In essence, the reputation of the Mayo Clinic pulls patients around the local physician and specialty referral network.

In reality, most organizations use a combination of push and pull strategies to control the channel of distribution. But it is essential in the development of marketing strategy to identify the intermediaries in the channel and to develop programs to control the flow of patients.

Promotion

The final element of marketing strategy is promotion. The promotional mix consists of four approaches: public relations, advertising, personal selling, and sales promotions.

In health care, reliance has traditionally been placed on public relations. Public relations can be defined as any nondirectly paid presentation or activity for an organization. PR activities consist of working with the media for the placement of favorable stories about the health care facilities or of the sponsoring community programs to create a favorable image of the group within the community. Health fairs, fun runs, and free blood pressure screening are all common activities that are designed to ultimately create a favorable impression.

A major function of public relations is to work to have favorable stories placed in the media about the health care group. Because the attention paid by the media is not directly paid for, a favorable story reported in the press about a doctor, a hospital, or an HMO is of great value. Most people view these stories as having a great deal of credibility. They are viewed differently from an ads. Yet it is in trying to obtain favorable press that the weakness of this approach is revealed. It is the rare physician who has not been interviewed by the media at some length. As most readers of this book can attest, reading an article in which you were interviewed often leads to a reaction such as, "I didn't say that." And, because publicity is a function of the media deciding to run the story, there is little control over the message. If the health care organization tries to get the story repeated on a second day, it is unlikely to be successful, because the media no longer view the story as newsworthy. It is because of these limitations that most health care organizations have turned to advertising.

Advertising can be defined as a directly paid form of presentation of a service, product, or organization. Because a health care organization pays the media to run its advertisement, the organization has control over several important elements. The health care organization can control *to whom* the message is sent, *when* the message is sent, *how often* the message is sent, and *how* the message is sent. The health care provider can decide what newspaper is best, what day of the week the ad should run, how large the ad should be, and how frequently the message should be told. None of these elements can be controlled in a story generated through public relations activities. A major limitation of advertising relative to public relations, however, involves credibility. Consumers understand an advertisement is a form of self-promotion and often process the information more critically.

While the purpose of this chapter is not to explain all the components of creating a successful advertising program, it is important to outline a few key ingredients. A well-run advertising campaign begins with a definition of the target audience. The organization should have a fairly well-defined profile of whom it wants to attract. In this way, the appropriate media can be selected to reach the target audience. Second, a well-run advertising campaign is centered around advertisements that are pretested with the intended audience. A major difference to date between many of the advertisements developed in health care, compared to more traditional companies, has been the lack of pretesting. Often, in health care organizations, an advertisement is developed internally and then placed with the media. The doctors in the group often review the ad and give approval or suggest some minor changes. In a well-run advertising campaign, the pretest should be conducted with a sample of people for whom the ad is intended. Do these people like the ad? Do they understand what is being said? Is there any additional information that they would like to see in the ad? These are the types of questions that are addressed in a pretest. Finally, in a well-run ad campaign, there is a measurable set of objectives that guide the copy and the media strategy of the campaign.

The third component of promotional strategy is the use of personal selling. Traditionally, salespeople were rare in health care organizations outside of HMOs, which had representatives who presented the respective plans within a company. Increasingly, however, the use of personal sales forces has grown for contact with intermediaries in the channel of distribution. Hospitals have used sales representatives to contact physicians; radiology departments have used salespeople to contact referral sources; and adolescent chemical dependency programs have salespeople contacting judges, social workers, and probation officers.[5]

Salespeople can perform multiple roles.[6] The common role is selling or obtaining new business. But salespeople are also useful in conducting field research on the competition or on prospective user needs. Salespeople also play an important missionary role of maintaining goodwill and of dealing with any user complaints or problems. For medical organizations that depend on referrals, this last role is particularly valuable.

The final component of promotional strategy involves the use of sales promotions, the common form being coupons. While a regular strategy for most consumer goods marketers, coupons have infrequently been used in health care. Some reported uses have been the offering of a free health screen for first-time users of a new service, or a small price reduction on the first office visit of a new patient. To a large extent, the value of sales promotions is the ability to track the response to an advertisement. Coupons allow the organization to track whether individuals are reading an ad and finding the offer of sufficient interest to act. In general, the response rate to direct mail coupons is one and one-half to three percent.

Summary

Marketing is a process that focuses on the buyers of a service. Essential to the development of any effective marketing strategy is the need to understand buyers' requirements and demands. Contrary to traditional health care planning, which is motivated by the requirements of those internal to the organization, marketing is an external to internal approach. After fully understanding buyers' requirements, the organization develops a strategy based on the four components of the marketing mix—product, price, place, and promotion.

References

1. For a comprehensive perspective on the nature of marketing and the role of consumer input, see Berkowitz, E., and others. *Marketing*. Third Edition. Homewood, Ill.: Richard D. Irwin, Inc., 1992, chap. 1.

2. An interesting article that displays the contribution of the marketing research approach is Tucker, L., and others. "The Role of Marketing Research in Securing a Certificate of Need for a New Renal Transplant Facility." *Journal of Health Care Marketing* 11(2):63-9, June 1991.

3. A detailed discussion of secondary data sources in health care is provided in Hillestad, S., and Berkowitz, E. *Health Care Marketing Plans: From Strategy to Action*. Second Edition. Rockville, Md.: Aspen Press, 1991, pp. 90-6.

4. A useful article to see the application of telephone interviewing is Gombeski, W., and others. "Overnight Assessment of Marketing Crises." *Journal of Health Care Marketing* 11(1):51-4, March 1991.

5. Bates, B., and McSurley, H. "The Sales Function in Radiology Departments." *Administrative Radiology* 8(9):16-9, Sept. 1989.

6. Mack, K., and Newbold, P. *Health Care Sales.* San Francisco, Calif.: Jossey-Bass Publishers, 1991, chap. 1.

Eric N. Berkowitz is Professor and Head, Department of Marketing, University of Massachusetts, Amherst.

CHAPTER 11

An Overview of Legal Issues

by Mark E. Lutes and Neil S. Olderman

Introduction

This chapter identifies certain legal concerns facing clinical department managers (CDMs). It is not intended to be a comprehensive or exhaustive discussion of all the potentially relevant issues. Rather, it is intended to familiarize CDMs with a number of the issues that may arise in the performance of their duties. Some of the topics discussed below may not be applicable to all CDMs. This would largely depend on the scope of the CDM's duties and the CDM's relationship with the particular health care organization. The chapter is divided into three parts. Each part identifies legal issues related to the roles typically assumed by CDMs within a health care organization—corporate director, peer reviewer, and patient care/quality assurance monitor.

Corporate Law Issues: The Corporate Director's Duties of Care and Loyalty

In some instances a member of a health care organization's clinical staff, oftentimes a medical staff officer or CDM, is elected to the organization's board of directors or is *ex officio* a member of the board by virtue of his or her position as a CDM. One purpose for including a member of the clinical staff on the board of directors is to have clinical staff representation and input in the organization's formulation of policy.

In such cases, a CDM's duties extend beyond merely representing the interests of fellow clinicians. Board members of a health care organization, like the members of any corporate board, are charged with the exercise of the duty of care and the duty of loyalty in performing their organizational functions. The functions of a board member are, among other things, to protect and preserve the corporation's financial solvency and stability; establish corporate governing policy; manage, supervise, and direct the affairs of the corporation; select competent officers; select competent and qualified clinical staff members; ensure the provision of care in accordance with prevailing quality standards; and avoid self-dealing or profiting unjustly from the relationship with the corporation. Each board function must be undertaken with that level of care that would be exercised by a reasonably prudent person with similar knowledge and experience under the circumstances. Moreover, such functions must be undertaken by the board member solely in the best interests of the corporation and not out of an interest in personal gain.

Until 1985, judicial interpretation of the duties of care and loyalty were characterized by the "business judgment rule." Under the business judgment rule courts found liability for breach of the duty of care only in cases of gross or willful negligence. Therefore, directors (or trustees in the case of a not-for-profit corporation) who took actions in good faith, after a reasonable effort had been made to become informed of the relevant issues, and who did not act in contravention of the organization's interests, were not saddled with liability for the unintended effects of their errors in judgment.

Some courts have begun to create a higher standard for directors in exercising their responsibilities. This new judicial thinking began with the Delaware Supreme Court's decision in *Smith v. Van Gorkom*.[1] Since the *Van Gorkom* decision, a line of cases has developed that stands for the proposition that directors will be held to a higher standard in determining whether they have met their fiduciary duties and hence are able to shield themselves from liability under the business judgment rule. One court has interpreted the duties of care and loyalty as requiring directors to take affirmative steps to defend and protect the interests with which they are entrusted.[2]

Some state legislatures have passed laws designed to offset the effects of these cases. The primary focus of such statutes is to expressly delineate the standards directors are to achieve in order to avoid liability. The statutes amount to codifications of the business judgment rule. In these jurisdictions, liability is not imposed in cases where there is no showing of willful or gross negligence on the part of the director. It would be prudent to become familiar with the expectations placed on directors by the law in your jurisdiction.

A breach of a director's duty of loyalty to the corporation occurs in cases where the director's personal interests and the best interests of the corporation are conflicting. Conflicts of interest typically arise where a director has some personal interest, usually economic, in the full board's taking certain actions. Transactions tainted by self-dealing may result in litigation against not only the organization and the interested director or trustee, but also the corporation's shareholders (or members in the case of a not-for-profit organization).

In cases where a conflict exists, the interested director must fully disclose his or her interest in the transaction and the decision must be made after fair and reasonable consideration, in an open manner and without fraud or imposition.[3] The interested director bears the burden of demonstrating that the transaction was fair from the corporation's perspective. Still, some states courts have held that in no case may a director or trustee profit from a transaction with the corporation that he or she serves, even if the corporation is provided beneficial terms.[4]

Medical Staff Credentialing and Peer Review Issues

It is not unlikely that, as an expert in a particular medical specialty or through familiarity with a particular case, a CDM will become part of a peer review program or a credentialing process. Therefore, knowledge of legal issues relating to credentialing and peer review could prevent potential liability on the part of the CDM and the health care organization.

Due Process

The principal grounds for judicial reversal of a health care organization's credentialing decision is whether the process itself was procedurally fair. The precise legal question asks whether adequate "due process" was afforded.

In the hospital setting, analysis of the due process issue is broken down into two major categories: due process afforded new applicants for staff privileges and due process afforded members of the medical staff whose privileges are under review. Traditionally, new applicants for staff privileges are deemed to have fewer due process rights, because, technically, nothing is being taken from them except an opportunity that the law considers a privilege as opposed to a right. A second subissue is whether the practitioner is seeking or has privileges at a public as opposed to a private institution. The answer to this question is similarly crucial in determining how much process is due.

Public institutions are considered agents of the state and as such must meet a higher standard of due process. The higher standard is imposed through the constitutional right to due process contained in the Fifth Amendment to the U.S. Constitution and made applicable to the states through the Fourteenth Amendment. Where a public institution is conducting the credentialing process, a more stringent standard will be applied in evaluating the due process afforded membership applicants and staff members. The courts in a majority of jurisdictions have been reluctant, however, to extend constitutional due process protections in the context of private hospital credentialing decisions.[5] Thus, for private hospitals, judicial review of credentialing decisions is generally confined to an inquiry as to whether the hospital followed its own bylaws.[6]

Some courts go so far as to deem the medical staff bylaws to be a contract between the hospital and the medical staff's members.[7]

In a few jurisdictions, the courts have looked beyond the procedure applied by a private hospital and reviewed the substance of the hospital's decision. New Jersey courts, for instance, have reasoned that the public interest in quality of care permits courts to determine if medical staff selections are not "arbitrary, capricious, or unreasonable." This approach was first enunciated in *Greisman v. Necomb Hosp.*,[8] and was based on findings that even private hospitals receive a substantial portion of their revenues from public funds, receive tax benefits, and often constitute virtual monopolies in their areas. California courts have applied common law fair process theory out of a concern that denial of medical staff membership would effectively impair the applicant's right to fully practice his or her profession.[9]

Immunity from Liability for Actions taken Incidental to the Credentialing and Peer Review Process Under the Health Care Quality Improvement Act
A principal concern among individuals taking part in the credentialing and peer review processes is whether they will be personally subject to civil claims brought by individuals alleging to have been harmed as a result of the decision or the process. A number of states have statutes protecting the participants in peer review actions. These state laws vary as to the activities and persons protected and therefore cannot be effectively discussed in this chapter. The statutory immunity is limited to certain peer review bodies and individuals defined in the statute to have assisted those bodies. Generally, peer review bodies engaged in the process of evaluating physician competence and quality of care or in any other activity delineated in the statute are granted immunity from suit where they adhere to appropriate standards or criteria in performing the review function.[10] Moreover, in 1986, Congress supplemented these state peer review immunity schemes with the Health Care Quality Improvement Act (HCQIA).[11] HCQIA provides a uniform federal scheme for immunity from civil suit to persons providing information to or performing the credentialing or peer review functions.

Under HCQIA's immunity provisions, persons who provide information to a health care entity,[12] its governing body, or any committee established by the health care entity to conduct professional review activities regarding the competence or professional conduct of a physician are immune from civil damages liability under state or and most federal law unless the person providing the information knowingly provides false information to the body performing professional review. However, the professional review body and persons assisting such bodies are protected from civil liability only in cases where the body's action is supported by the presence of the following four conditions:

✦ The body reasonably believed that taking such action would further the provision of high-quality health care.

✦ A reasonable effort was made by the body to obtain the facts of the matter.

✦ The practitioner was afforded adequate notice and hearing as part of the professional review process.

✦ The body reasonably believed the action taken was warranted in light of the facts presented.

The immunity provided professional review activities under HCQIA does not apply to actions brought under the federal civil rights laws, injunctive or declaratory judgment actions, actions brought by governmental agencies, or criminal suits. Similarly, actions brought by nonphysician practitioners or chiropractors do not fall within the scope of HCQIA's immunity protections.

In addition, states were given the option to prohibit the use of HCQIA immunity for actions brought under state law. The deadline for "opting in" or "opting out" was October 14, 1989. Some states have elected to "opt out" and expand due process rights for physicians. California was one state that selected this alternative course. The effect of a state "opting out" is to force professional review bodies to offer a panoply of fair process protections as part of their decision making process. Moreover, immunity would not be guaranteed even in cases where all due process requirements imposed by state law were met. As of September 1, 1990, HCQIA requires the reporting of certain adverse actions taken against the clinical privileges of physicians to the medical licensing board.[13] Those adverse actions that must be reported include:

✦ Any action taken by the health care entity that adversely affects the clinical privileges of a physician for longer than 30 days.

✦ An action that results in the physician's surrender of his or her clinical privileges while the physician's competence or professional conduct are being investigated by the health care entity's professional review body.

✦ The surrender of clinical privileges in return for an investigation not taking place.

By law, the report must be filed with the state licensing board within 15 days of the date on which the adverse action is taken. The state licensing board then has 15 days to file a report with the U.S. Secretary of Health and Human Services, the agency charged with the development of the National Practitioner Data Bank. Further, the state licensing board must inform the Secretary of a health care entity's failure to file a required report. HCQIA also provides protection to persons and entities making the required reports without knowledge of their falsity.

Furthermore, HCQIA indirectly imposes a duty on health care entities to search the National Practitioner Data Bank prior to making any credentialing or recredentialing decision. Failure to inquire into a practitioner's file, although not expressly penalized in the statute, could expose the health care entity to the risk of having such a failure used as *prima facie* evidence of negligence in an action for negligent hiring or retention of a clinical staff member, because HCQIA provides that the health care facility is presumed to know all relevant information in the Data Bank. Therefore, in an effort to reduce the risks of exposure to liability, CDMs should be aware of their roles in the credentialing and peer review processes and, where appropriate, make efforts to ensure that proper Data Bank reporting and inquiry are a regular practice of the health care organization.

Patient Care Issues

Nondiscrimination in the Provision of Care
Federal Law. There are a number of federal statutes that require certain health care institutions to provide health care services on a nondiscriminatory basis.

Further, the Constitution, as well as state and local laws, impose a similar legal mandate. More specifically, the Civil Rights Act of 1964[14] prohibits discrimination based on race in designated places of "public accommodation" and by publicly owned facilities. The provisions contained in Titles II and IV have been applied by the courts to public hospitals. Additionally, Title VI of the Civil Rights Act prohibits discrimination on the basis of race, color, or national origin by an institution receiving "federal financial assistance." Hospitals receiving Medicare and/or Medicaid funds are deemed to be recipients of federal financial assistance. Accordingly, the nondiscrimination requirement is applied to the hospital's admission policies, the availability of services, and the assignment of rooms.

A second federal statute, the Hill-Burton Act,[15] requires that hospitals receiving assistance under the Hill-Burton program make their facilities available to all persons within the community. This community service requirement is agreed to by the hospital as a condition to its receiving federal funds. Hospitals receiving Hill-Burton funds are required to participate in the Medicare/ Medicaid programs; provide emergency care to persons residing or employed in the service area without regard to their ability to pay; and make hospital services available to persons within the community without regard to race, creed, color, or national origin or to whether their treating physician is a physician on staff at the hospital. Under the Hill-Burton Act, it is also the hospital's duty to ensure that physicians on its medical staff agree to accept Medicaid patients.

A Hill-Burton hospital must not only generally agree to make services available to the community, but also guarantee a specified volume of free care. The "uncompensated care" assurance is calculated as an amount of free care equal to 10 percent of the Hill-Burton assistance granted under the Act or 3 percent of the hospital's Medicare/Medicaid operating costs. This free care assurance must be upheld for a period of 20 years. In the event a hospital is unable to meet its free care obligation for a given year, the amount of free care is carried forward to the following year. In cases where a particular hospital is unable to meet its free-care obligations, the hospital must establish out-reach programs to satisfy the terms of the Hill-Burton Act grant. The Department of Health and Human Services, Public Health Service, Office of Facilities Compliance, enforces the Hill-Burton Act.

The courts have held that a patient may bring a private right of action to enforce a hospital's free-care obligation under the Act.[16] Nevertheless, hospitals are not required to render free care in cases where they do not have the necessary facilities or where they reject a patient's transfer absent knowledge of the existence of emergency circumstances.[17]

A third federal statute, the Rehabilitation Act of 1973, prohibits discrimination in federally assisted programs against persons who have a handicap condition or have a record of such impairment or are perceived as having a handicap impairment. The United States Supreme Court has interpreted the term "handicap" to include a communicable disease such as tuberculosis.[18] Commentators suggest that this rationale is likely to be construed by the courts as including AIDS and AIDS-Related Conditions (ARC) within the scope of the term handicap for purposes of the Rehabilitation Act of 1973.

Several states have adopted analogous statutes. Some jurisdictions have gone so far as to expressly hold AIDS as being a handicap under the local law.[19] The Rehabilitation Act of 1973 provides for a private right of action to enforce the nondiscrimination provision contained in Section 504 of the Act.

From a constitutional perspective, the due process and equal protection clauses of the Fourteenth Amendment to the United States Constitution are applicable to public hospitals. The Fourteenth Amendment provides that "no state shall deprive any person of life, liberty, or property without due process of law, nor deny any person within its jurisdiction the equal protection of the laws." In the public hospital setting, the Fourteenth Amendment has been used successfully by individuals seeking care at a particular hospital.

Nevertheless, the definition of public hospital has taken on a life of its own. The public/private question is at issue, because the Fourteenth Amendment is only applicable to "state action" as opposed to private actions. This gives rise to a question as to whether a private hospital can ever be engaged in action sufficient to constitute state action. On the one hand, there is the argument that, if a private facility accepts state or federal funds, it is in fact engaged in state action. In general, however, a hospital's participation in the Medicare/Medicaid program, the grant of a federal or state tax exemption, and the acceptance of governmental financial aid have been found to be insufficient to convert a private hospital's actions or policies into actions of the state.

There are, however, limited circumstances in which private hospitals may be so intertwined with a public or governmental responsibility that the courts will find the presence of state action for purposes of applying the Constitution. For example, the Fourth Circuit has held that private hospitals participating in the Hill-Burton program were engaged in state action based on the fact that they cooperated in a federal-state planning function and were receiving funds as a result.[20] Furthermore, a hospital located on land in which a local government had a future interest conditioned on the hospital's ceasing its operations and which received local governmental financial assistance was held to be engaged in state action for purposes of the Fourteenth Amendment.[21]

State Law. Both state and local law may require nondiscrimination in the provision of services. Such laws are generally applied to business entities serving the public or providing public accommodations. Depending on a particular statute, such nondiscrimination provisions may be applicable to private hospitals. Typically, these nondiscrimination requirements will appear in the hospital licensure statutes. Such nondiscrimination requirements may also appear in state tax-exemption laws, as is the case in Oklahoma. Some of these state or local laws impose nondiscrimination provisions that are atypical in that they are applicable to categories other than race, religion, color, national origin, sex, age, or handicap. These nondiscrimination provisions prohibit hospitals from discriminating in providing services to or admitting patients of physicians who do not have staff privileges at the particular hospital.

Montana has such a nondiscrimination requirement. The language in the statute is broader than the typical nondiscrimination provision in that it cuts across racial lines and is not limited to express classifications set forth in the statute. From the patient's perspective, the Montana statute is easier to litigate under. Instead of having to prove that there was some racial, ethnic, or sex-based rationale for not being admitted or treated properly, a patient is able to make the same charges based primarily on the fact that he or she was not referred to the facility by a member of its medical staff.

Detention of Patients

CDMs may encounter situations in which a patient is admitted to a facility against his or her wishes. In some cases, a CDM may be given oversight responsibilities in this area that would include the monitoring of staff compliance with a hospital's or health care organization's patient detention policy.

Patients admitted and treated in facilities against their wishes have traditionally sued the facility on the basis of false imprisonment. In short, any patient held against his or her will and without legal authority has a cause of action against the party causing the nonconsensual detention. In false imprisonment cases, actual restraint does not have to be proven. The courts have held that threats by medical or hospital staff, which would lead a reasonable person to fear harm, provide sufficient restraint to maintain an action based on false imprisonment. Similarly, detaining a patient for failure to pay an outstanding hospital bill has been deemed to constitute false imprisonment.

State statutes may be instructive in delineating explicit conditions under which detention of patients is permitted and procedures for instituting such detentions. For example, New York's Patient Bill of Rights statute[22] explicitly states the conditions under which a patient may be restrained either physically or through the use of chemicals. All states have laws providing specific procedures for committing an individual who is mentally ill or a dangerous substance abuser to a mental health or substance abuse treatment facility. Generally, hospitals are permitted to detain these individuals in the course of treatment upon notifying the appropriate authorities and obtaining commitment or custody orders from such authority.

Discharge Planning

Assuming a patient has been admitted to a hospital, has been treated without being unlawfully detained, and is medically ready for discharge, the hospital must then satisfy its posthospital care obligations. Generally, the hospital is not obligated from a legal perspective to provide posthospital care or ensure that the plan of posthospital care is actually implemented. The hospital is merely required to assess the patient's medical status at the time of discharge, identify posthospital services that may benefit the patient, and make a reasonable effort to make those services available to the patient. In cases where the hospital demonstrates a lack of due care in performing the discharge planning function, liability will be imposed. In cases where there was a clear failure to inform the patient of a reasonably foreseeable outcome of discharge or where the hospital failed to ascertain the patient's circumstances relative to planning post-discharge care, courts have found negligence on the part of the hospital.

In certain cases, patients will refuse to leave the hospital upon notification from a physician that they are ready for discharge. Depending on his or her specific authority, a CDM could find him- or herself in the middle of a dispute between the patient and the treating physician. In some states, the statutes are instructive as to the ramifications of a patient's failure to leave a hospital. For example, North Carolina law makes it a misdemeanor for a patient to fail to leave a hospital upon the discharge order of two physicians. In the event that state law is silent on the issue, the hospital may resort to an action to evict the patient as a trespasser. At least one court has suggested that a hospital has a duty to take such action in the interests of other members of the community desirous of using the hospital's limited resources.[23]

Patient "Antidumping" Requirements

Beginning in 1986, Congress required hospitals participating in the Medicare program to provide examinations and treatment to individuals with emergency medical conditions in an effort to prevent refusal of treatment or transferring of individuals to other facilities before instituting emergency medical treatment because the individual lacked the financial resources to pay for the emergency services. This federal law is commonly referred to as COBRA or patient "antidumping" legislation.[24,25] The antidumping law is of particular interest to CDMs in the emergency medicine area. However, it is prudent for every CDM, no matter what the area of specialty, to be familiar with the rules regarding treatment and transfer of emergency patients, because a variety of clinical departments may be involved in the treatment of emergency patients.

Basic Screening Requirement. The patient antidumping law is applicable to any hospital that participates in the Medicare program.[26] Further, such provisions apply to any physician who provides services at a hospital that is required to comply with COBRA and who is in a position to examine, treat, or transfer individuals presenting themselves at the hospital who would otherwise be entitled to the protections of the antidumping laws.

The basic requirements of COBRA are that the Medicare-participating hospital screen the condition of any person who seeks treatment in its emergency department to determine whether an emergency medical condition exists.[26,27] The duty to screen the condition of any person applies to individuals seeking services from a Medicare-participating hospital whether or not the individual is covered by Medicare or has the ability to pay for such services. As a practical matter, a screening examination may not be delayed in order to determine the individual's method of payment or type of insurance.[28]

If an emergency medical condition exists, the individual must be given treatment in order to stabilize the condition prior to being transferred to another facility.[29] In the event the hospital is unable to stabilize the emergency medical condition, the statute imposes specific requirements before a transfer may be made.

In order to fulfill the hospital's duties under the statute, persons in an emergency department must conduct an appropriate screening examination within the capabilities of the department to determine whether an emergency medical condition exists.[30] This means that all resources routinely available to the emergency department, including ancillary services, must be accessible and usable in the initial screening process.[30]

If an emergency medical condition exists, the hospital must provide either further examination and treatment within its capabilities to stabilize the medical condition, unless such treatment is refused by the patient, or an appropriate transfer to another health care facility. COBRA does not require that treatment be provided if the individual or surrogate refuses to consent to treatment or refuses to be transferred to another facility where treatment could be provided, assuming that transfer would be appropriate.[31] Nevertheless, a hospital is required to take all reasonable steps to secure the individual's written and informed consent refusing an examination and treatment or refusing a transfer.

Consent Rule and Certification of Transfer. If the hospital is unable to obtain informed consent from the individual refusing an examination and/or treatment, it should carefully document the specific events leading up to such refusal and the ultimate failure to examine or treat the individual. This is important because, under COBRA, it is presumed that the individual presenting him- or herself at an emergency department is requesting examination and treatment for a medical condition. The burden is on the hospital to establish by a preponderance of the evidence that the request for such examination for treatment was withdrawn.[32]

An individual whose emergency medical condition has not been stabilized may be transferred from the hospital under certain conditions, including whether the transfer is both "authorized" and "appropriate." The transfer is authorized only if it is made with the individual's informed consent or with a physician's certification and is appropriate.

COBRA requires that the hospital take all reasonable steps to obtain evidence of informed consent. Emergency department physicians must be prepared to inform the individual or a surrogate of the risks and/or benefits of a transfer or a lack of transfer in order to obtain written informed consent.[33] In the event the individual or his or her surrogate is unable to provide informed consent, the transfer of an individual whose medical condition has not been stabilized may be based on a physician's certification.

The physician certification essentially states that, based upon the information available at the time, the medical benefits reasonably expected from medical treatment at the transferee facility outweigh the increased risks to the individual due to the transfer.[34] Under COBRA only a physician may currently certify a transfer. Effective July 1, 1990, hospitals were required to designate on-call physicians to be responsible for making a risk/benefit determination regarding whether a transfer is appropriate.

In the event no physician is physically present at the hospital, the hospital must ensure that a physician is available for consultation and that the physician is the person who determines that the transfer is appropriate. Designated physicians who fail to respond to a request for certification of transfer are potentially subject to civil action and statutory penalties.

Physician certification of a transfer must always include the physician's signature and should be obtained at the earliest possible time. COBRA permits, under certain emergency circumstances, the communication of a physician certification via telephone. However, a physician's signature is always required and must be obtained at the earliest possible time.

Other Transfer Prerequisites. In order for a patient transfer to be appropriate, certain conditions must be met in addition to obtaining either a patient consent or physician certification, whichever is applicable.[35] The requisite conditions are that:

✦ Medical treatment, within the capabilities of the emergency department of the transferring facility, has been provided in order to minimize the health risks to the individual.

✦ The transferee facility must have consented to receive the individual and must have available space and qualified personnel to treat the individual.

✦ All available medical records that relate to the individual's emergency medical condition and that include observations of the individual's condition, preliminary diagnosis, treatment provided, results of tests administered, and the informed written consent for the transfer or physician certification if applicable must be presented to the transferee hospital upon transfer.

✦ The transfer must be conducted by qualified personnel and through the use of transportation equipment that is most appropriate in light of the individual's medical condition.

HCFA has taken the position in the past that transferring hospitals must complete the transfer of patients to transferee facilities even in cases where the transferee facility refuses to accept the transfer because of lack of capacity. HCFA staff members have found in the past that the receiving facility will make space available somehow upon the transfer of the individual. This policy statement may be indicative of HCFA's lack of tolerance for institutions that refuse transfers on the basis of capacity.

Enforcement. The requirements of the patient antidumping statute may be enforced by HCFA, a transferee facility, or the individual suffering harm because of a violation of the antidumping law. In cases where HCFA enforces the provisions of the antidumping law, it will typically order the state agency responsible for ensuring that the hospital complies with Medicare requirements to conduct an investigation. Assuming the state agency's investigation determines there is a violation, HCFA may recommend termination of the Medicare provider agreement at the end of a 90-day waiting period. The decision regarding the determination and timing of the Medicare provider agreement is made by the HCFA regional office with jurisdiction over the facility.

In the event HCFA determines that a violation of COBRA has occurred, it may seek to assess civil monetary penalties through an action filed by the Office of the Inspector General (OIG). The law is unclear as to whether the civil penalties contemplated by COBRA would be available to a party other than the Secretary of Health and Human Services. At least one federal court has held that it has jurisdiction to hear a claim for civil penalties brought by an individual against a physician for allegedly violating COBRA.[36]

Civil monetary penalties may be imposed against the hospital or the physician. The OIG may impose civil penalties of up to $50,000 per violation.[37] However, the civil monetary penalty assessable against a hospital with fewer than 100 beds is limited to $25,000. The civil monetary penalties are in addition to suspension or termination of the participation agreement with Medicare.

A physician who is responsible for the screening examination and other necessary treatment may be assessed civil monetary penalties if he or she knowingly violates a requirement of COBRA.[38] The penalties are capped at $50,000 per violation. The penalties apply to physicians who sign a certification to transfer an individual if the physician knew or should have known that the benefits of the transfer did not outweigh its risks. Moreover, civil penalties may be assessed against a physician who misrepresents an individual's conditions or the obligations of the health care facility. In addition, the physician may be excluded from participation under Medicare if it is found that his or her violation of COBRA was knowing and willful or negligent.

A hospital as well as an on-call physician may be subject to liability for a violation of COBRA in the event the on-call physician refuses to or fails to appear to provide stabilizing treatment to the patient.[39] The penalties would not apply to a physician who orders the transfer of an individual because the physician determines that, without the services of an on-call physician, the benefits of a transfer outweigh the apparent risks.[39] Therefore, even where a hospital does not knowingly violate the provisions of COBRA, it still may be subject to liability for the acts of its agents and the physician through whom it looks to satisfy its COBRA responsibilities. Furthermore, a facility that suffers economic loss as a result of an individual who is improperly transferred is entitled to seek restitution from the hospital transferring the individual.[40]

Finally, COBRA provides a private right of action to individuals suffering personal harm as a direct result of a hospital's violation of COBRA. Such individuals are permitted to pursue damages available under state law for such injuries or such other equitable relief as is appropriate.[41] The statutory private right of action and claims are against the hospital and not the physician. However, the physician may be subject to medical malpractice claims brought by the individual injured by the physician's negligence in treatment.

Administrative Requirements for Facilities. COBRA imposes on the hospital several administrative requirements. First, the hospital must adopt a policy to ensure compliance with the antidumping provisions of COBRA. This is also a requirement of the Joint Commission on Accreditation of Healthcare Organizations (JCAHO). JCAHO requires that, as a condition of accreditation, the hospital have an established policy regarding the treatment of individuals in its emergency department. Generally, a hospital's antidumping policy includes a statement of intent; the pertinent statutory definitions; the hospital's method for coordinating the services of the various hospital departments that may be required to comply with the terms of the policy, including the emergency department, the labor and delivery department, and those ancillary service departments that render services to the emergency department; the responsibilities of on-call physicians and the consequences of failing to respond; the requirements of transferring an individual; the procedures or requirements necessary to determine if the facility lacks the capacity to accept a transfer; the identification of persons responsible for making any necessary decisions; the requirement that the treating physicians obtain and document the individual's consent to transfer; and the hospital's policy with regard to retention of the records of patients treated and/or transferred under the COBRA requirements.

Hospitals are required to maintain medical records and other records related to individuals who are transferred to or from a facility prior to stabilizing an emergency medical condition. The records are to be kept for a period of five years from the date of the transfer. COBRA also specifies the required contents of the medical records. One key aspect of the patient transfer record is the patient consent form or, in the alternative, the physician certification form.

COBRA requires a hospital to maintain a list of physicians who are on-call to provide medical treatment required to stabilize individuals with emergency medical conditions. The hospital must also post signs conspicuously throughout the emergency department that specify the rights of an individual to receive medical treatment. In addition, hospitals are required to post signs indicating whether or not the hospital participates in the Medicaid program under a state plan approved under Medicare. HCFA has issued detailed and specific instructions regarding the posting of the notice and the form of the notice.

Analogous State Law. Over the past several years, various states have begun to enact antidumping legislation. Numerous states including California, New York, Florida and Texas have enacted laws to guarantee access to emergency care and to prohibit the denial of services. As is the case in Florida, several state anti-dumping laws allow for the denial, revocation, or suspension of a license for hospitals found to violate the emergency services requirements. A patient dumping incident, in many states, could threaten both a hospital's state licensure and its Medicare participation. Further, because the federal statute does not preempt state law in the area, HCFA and the state department of health could arguably proceed concurrently, and sanctions could be triggered at both levels.

Patient Consent to Treatment

In recent years, the issues surrounding a patient's consent to treatment have taken on new importance. The right of the patient to control the course of his or her medical treatment, including the right to terminate care, has become a prevalent issue in hospitals around the country. The requirements for patient consent are now being imposed through statutory/regulatory mandates rather than through common law. It is important that a CDM, and the providers under his or her charge, understand the rules for communicating and decision-making present in every patient/physician relationship not only for purposes of reducing the risk of potential liability, but also as a means of improving patient satisfaction.

Consent and Informed Consent Compared. Consent encompasses two separate doctrines, consent and informed consent. Under the doctrine of consent, a physician is required to obtain the patient's permission prior to beginning treatment. The failure of the physician to obtain consent constitutes the tort of battery.[42] Battery, in tort law, is nonconsensual touching. Therefore, motive, including a desire to protect the patient, is irrelevant, as is the fact that the treatment may have been administered appropriately.

Civil actions for battery based on a failure to obtain consent are most likely to be brought as a result of a physician's providing treatment other than that described to the patient or altering the method of delivery of particular treatment without informing the patient.[43] Consent need not always be expressed. It can be implied from the patient's conduct, as is often the case with routine medical procedures.

Informed consent doctrine was developed by the courts in cases brought against providers under negligence law and is not applicable in cases involving the intentional tort of battery. In order to establish a prima facie case of negligence, the plaintiff must establish that a duty was owed by the allegedly negligent defendant; such duty was breached; and such breach caused actual injury to the plaintiff. The theory of informed consent is based on the principle that a physician stands in a special relationship of trust toward a patient. The physician owes the patient the duty not to withhold any facts that are necessary to form the basis of an intelligent decision by the patient to undergo the proposed treatment.[44]

During the 1970s, many states adopted informed consent statutes that generally codified the common law consent requirements, often adopting the professional practice standards for disclosure.

Scope of Disclosure. The principal issue in informed consent cases is the scope of the physician's explanation. Generally, the courts have required that a patient be told the nature and purpose of the procedure, the risks and consequences, the alternatives to the proposed course of treatment, and, most recently, the risks of no treatment at all.

In recognition of the fact that certain information must be provided, it appears that at least two standards have emerged with respect to how much information need be disclosed to the patient. One standard is the "professional practice standard," which requires the physician to make such disclosure as a reasonable medical practitioner in similar circumstances would make.[45] In practical terms, the professional practice standard is proved in court through the use of expert testimony as to the applicable standard in the community.

An alternative standard is the "reasonable patient" or "materiality rule," which requires the physician to disclose the information that a reasonable person in the patient's position would consider material in deciding whether to undergo the proposed treatment.[46] Under the reasonable patient rule, the determination as to whether the detail of the disclosure was sufficient is made by a jury as opposed to an expert witness. As a general rule, however, the disclosure of a particular risk in large part depends on the frequency and the severity of the risk. Very severe risks, such as death, damage to physical appearance or sexual functioning, and likelihood of incapacitation are considered material and subject to disclosure even if they are rare.

Patients alleging a lack of informed consent must prove not only that the physician breached his or her duty to provide adequate information to make a decision, but also that the patient would not have consented if he or she had known the risks and that the patient was injured by a risk that was not disclosed.

Exceptions to the Consent Requirement. Several exceptions have been created by the courts to the general rule that consent must be obtained prior to performing certain medical procedures. One exception is in the case of an emergency. Generally, this is found to mean that, if the delay in treatment necessary to obtain the patient consent would result in significant harm to the patient, the physician may proceed with treatment without consent.[47] At least one court has held that the treatment being provided without consent need not be life-saving as long as time is critical and the potential harm to the patient is more than trivial. However, where it is possible to obtain consent from a patient's appropriate surrogate, such consent should be obtained, even in an emergency.[48]

Another exception to the general rule of consent is in cases where a patient is under general anesthesia in surgery and an unanticipated condition arises that the physician determines requires attention in order to protect the patient from the risk and the discomfort of a second surgical procedure.[49] The condition must truly be unanticipated in order to fall within the exception. The courts have not been quick to find a condition to be unanticipated if it results in a procedure to

171

remove an organ or alter reproductive capacity or that significantly increases the risks associated with a particular surgery. However, in cases where a physician discusses the possibility that an unanticipated condition might arise during surgery prior to actually performing the surgery, courts are more likely to find in favor of the physician under the exception.[50]

A third exception to the general rule of consent is in cases involving a therapeutic privilege. The therapeutic privilege may be invoked where a physician reasonably believes that the patient's mental or physical well-being would suffer as a result of the physician's disclosure of certain information in order to obtain the patient's consent.

Finally, the patient may request that he or she not be informed. This is more commonly known as waiver of informed consent.

Hospital Policy Development. The consent issue is particularly important to CDMs, because hospitals have been held liable in cases where physicians fail to obtain consent, even where the physician is not an employee. Additionally, JCAHO requires hospitals to develop and implement informed consent policies. State hospital licensing departments may also regulate informed consent policies and practices. At least one court has suggested that hospitals may have an affirmative duty to require physicians to make proper disclosure to their patients.[51] Furthermore, studies have shown that consent policies enhance communication between staff and patients and may improve patient satisfaction.

An effective consent policy should contain a requirement that the physician obtain the patient's consent. Responsibility for obtaining patient consent should not be delegated by the physician to nurses, interns, or residents. Consent should be obtained through a conversation between the physician and the patient. The physician's explanation of the risks and the procedures should be in language that a layman can understand. Further, in the case of non-English speaking patients, translations should be provided.

The physician should inform the patient of the nature and purpose of the procedure or treatment, the risks, the alternatives, and the risks of no treatment at all. Most important, the patient should be given an opportunity to ask questions. Finally, the patient should be informed about the individual performing the procedure or surgery.

Consent should be obtained prior to the proposed treatment to provide the patient with adequate time to deliberate. However, consent should not be sought so far in advance as to allow the patient's physical condition to change. If possible, consent should be obtained under circumstances in which the patient's ability to absorb the information and make a rational decision is not effected, as might be the case where the patient is in severe pain or under sedation.

Moreover, the informed consent policy should define mental capacity and specify the surrogates authorized to act in the event the patient is found to lack mental capacity. A psychiatric evaluation should be recommended in the case where a patient's mental capacity is unclear. Finally, the policy should include a procedure to obtain patient consent where the patient has no surrogate.

Some states have enacted statutory requirements for disclosure that mandate that certain risks be disclosed by the physician and that certain procedures be followed in informing patients. Generally, the courts seem to strictly adhere to the standards set out in the statute when hearing cases alleging failure to properly disclose.

Patient Refusal of Treatment

The law governing the right to refuse or discontinue medical treatment is predominantly a creature of the states. The judicial opinions in this area reveal the presence of two conflicting principles. The first principle is the notion that a mentally competent adult patient has the right to refuse treatment. This principle is grounded in the notion that each man is considered to be the master of his own body and, assuming he is mentally capable to make such a decision, may expressly prohibit the performance of life-saving surgery or other medical treatment.[52] The second principle is that medical care necessary to preserve life must be provided, absent some recognized legal exception. The courts have derived this rule from the emergency exception to the informed consent rule and from the traditional paternalistic role the courts play with respect to medical treatment for incompetent persons.[53]

Competent Adults. Competent adults have been held to have a qualified right to refuse medical treatment, including life-sustaining treatment, based on a right to privacy and on religious grounds.[54] Furthermore, the courts have recognized a patient's right to refuse medical treatment based on a common law right of self-determination and on public policy grounds.[55] However, the competent adult patient's right to self-determination is limited. The courts have recognized four countervailing interests relative to the patient's right of self-determination: preservation of life, protection of the interests of innocent third parties, prevention of suicide, and protection of the ethical integrity of the medical profession.

Previous judicial determinations have been based primarily on preservation of life and/or protection of the interests of innocent third parties. Typically, the state's interest in preservation of life is offset in cases where a terminally ill patient is receiving prolonged medical care that is determined to result in extending the patient's suffering. However, in *Cruzan v. Director*,[56] the U.S. Supreme Court held that the state's interest in preservation of life necessarily requires a greater level of proof of a patient's desire to terminate life-sustaining treatment. Along these lines, various states have begun to enact living will statutes in an attempt to create a legal avenue for the proof of a patient's wishes in the event of terminal illness that could be used as evidence probative of the patient's intent.

In cases involving refusal of treatment based on religious beliefs, the courts generally apply more restrictive standards, particularly if there are third-party interests involved, such as unborn or minor children. For example, the courts have routinely ordered blood transfusions for pregnant women or mothers of small children despite contrary religious beliefs.[57] However, there is a minority of cases that reject the majority view.[58]

Incompetent Adults. The incompetent patient's right to self-determination has been upheld on a variety of grounds in cases where there is a medical consensus that the patient is terminally ill and without hope of recovery.[59] The U.S. Supreme Court has held that, in cases where an incompetent patient is not terminally ill, even where they are in a permanent vegetative state, the state's interest in preserving life supersedes the patient's interest in privacy or self-determination, as well as the presumptive guardianship rights of the patient's family.

In cases involving legally or mentally incompetent patients, the issue comes down to whether a decision as to the patient's well-being can be made by some other party, who is called the surrogate decision-maker. There is a rebuttable presumption that the family of a legally or mentally incompetent patient is an appropriate surrogate for purposes of exercising the patient's rights. However, the Supreme Court recently added another wrinkle to the rebuttable presumption standard. In *Cruzan*,[59] the Court recognized the state's interest in preserving life. The Court concluded that there is no constitutional requirement for a state to recognize family relationships where the family intends to act contrary to the interests of the state and there is no other probative evidence supporting the patient's desire to refuse treatment. The five-member majority of the Supreme Court ultimately held that the state can require "clear and convincing" evidence of the patient's desire to refuse treatment based on the court's rationale that incompetent persons do not possess the same rights as competent persons because they are unable to make an informed and voluntary choice to exercise those rights.

Parents as Surrogates for Minors. The law is slightly different with regard to the rights of parents acting as surrogate decision-makers on behalf of their minor children. A majority of the courts have prohibited parents and legal guardians from refusing life-sustaining care for their minor children, especially in cases where there is a consensus that the prognosis with treatment is favorable.[60] Some state legislatures have mandated that parents of minors provide medically necessary care for their children even if such care is contrary to the parents' religious beliefs.[61]

Further, several courts have ordered parents to provide medically necessary care for their children where the court determines that the failure to do so poses an unreasonable risk of harm to the child even in cases where such care is contrary to the parents' religious beliefs.[62] However, parents and legal guardians have been permitted by the courts to decline certain conventional medical treatments in favor of unorthodox approaches.[63] Where there is medical consensus that a minor is terminally ill or in a persistent vegetative state and that treatment would be futile or inadvisable, the withholding of such treatment has been permitted.[64] In cases involving mature minors, the courts have occasionally permitted the minor to refuse certain treatments on religious grounds.[65] For newborn children with severe disabilities that would cause death if left untreated, the courts have gone both ways.[66]

Congress and some state legislatures have acted to fill the void left by the lack of consensus among the courts. Today, there are federal and state statutes that establish standards for the withholding of medical treatment in the case of minors. The federal statute[67] permits withholding of treatment where the child is chronically and irreversibly comatose, treatment would merely prolong dying, or treatment otherwise would be futile or inhumane.

Nutrition and hydration must be provided in all cases under the federal law. The decision to withdraw or withhold nutrition or hydration by artificial means has been held to be governed by the same principles applied in cases involving the withdrawal of medical treatment. The Supreme Court, in *Cruzan*,[59] espoused this view, although the issue was not directly before the Court. The California Court of Appeals quashed an attempted criminal indictment of two physicians who withdrew an artificial feeding tube from a vegetative patient in accordance with the wishes of the patient's family.[68] The Court's reasoning in this case was based on the grounds that artificial nutrition was indistinguishable from other medical treatments.

Confidentiality of Medical Records and Patient Information
The right of physical possession and control of a patient's medical record is vested in the provider. Possession and control of documents related to the patient's treatment, such as x-rays, laboratory reports, and consultants' reports, are similarly vested in the provider. Neither the patient nor his or her authorized representative has a right to physical possession of the medical record. However, the right to possess and control the physical record is distinguished in the law from the right to control access to the information contained in the record. Generally, patients and legitimately interested third parties have the right, under certain circumstances, to inspect and copy the record and/or to receive certain information contained in the record.

Technically, there is no constitutional right of privacy. However, the U.S. Supreme Court has inferred the right to privacy from the Fifth and Fourteenth Amendments to the Constitution.[69] Generally, the right has not been extended specifically to confidentiality of information. The Supreme Court has, however, suggested the existence of a constitutional right to preserve confidentiality relative to medical treatment that is vested in every patient.[70] In addition, some lower federal courts and state courts have found a constitutional right to privacy in cases involving disclosure of medical information.[71] Nonetheless, the patient's constitutional right to privacy with respect to disclosure of information in his or her medical records has not been recognized in all situations. For example, one court has held that the disclosure of the names of abortion clinic patients was not violative of the patient's constitutional right to privacy.[72]

There are several federal and state statutes that protect the confidentiality of Medicare records, alcohol and drug abuse records of patients treated in a federally assisted program or activity relating to alcoholism/drug abuse, medical records maintained by federal agencies, confidential information contained in peer review organization records, and information contained in mental health research records that identifies research subjects. Further, the confidentiality of medical records has been established by statute and regulation in several states. However, a majority of states continue to rely on common law, ethical standards, and professional norms to protect the confidentiality of patient information. In states where statutory protection is provided, the laws generally require that the disclosing party obtain the patient's consent prior to releasing or transferring patient medical records.[73]

In addition to record protection statutes or case law, many states have physician/patient privilege statutes that apply to physician testimony as opposed to the disclosure of confidential medical information contained in a record. The courts have generally construed the statutory privilege narrowly to apply to in-court testimony of a physician because patient privilege did not exist at common law but was developed by statute. Physicians and hospitals are not permitted to waive the privilege nor are they permitted to assert the privilege on their own behalf. The privilege is asserted solely on the patient's behalf. Some courts have held that a hospital or a physician has a duty to assert the physician/patient privilege when records are sought in a court proceeding.

In cases where a patient brings a personal injury suit against a provider, the physician/patient privilege is waived.[74] In addition, various state legislatures have adopted statutes protecting communications between certain providers— i.e., psychotherapists-patient privilege statutes—and the confidentiality of information contained in records such as those prepared as a result of treatment in a mental health facility or in an alcohol and drug abuse program.

As for professional standards governing the confidentiality of medical records, the JCAHO medical record standards require written consent of the patient or an authorized representative as a condition to the release of medical information to persons not otherwise authorized to receive the information.[75] Similarly, the *Underlying Principles of Medical Ethics* of the American Medical Association[76] and the *Patient's Bill of Rights* of the American Hospital Association[77] require that patient confidences be safeguarded in accordance with relevant law.

Patient Access. Many states have enacted statutes and regulations that grant patients and/or their authorized representatives access to their medical records. Generally, these statutes include a provision permitting a patient to inspect the record itself, as well as to know the information contained therein. Some states have enacted statutes that limit patient access to their own psychiatric records. These statutes typically do not address access to records by minors. Minors have been permitted access to their medical record in cases where they are legally recognized as being capable of consenting to treatment.

Several courts have recognized a patient's common law right to access to his or her medical records. However, such access is limited in cases where the information contained in the medical record would be detrimental to the interests of the patient, a third party, or the custodian of the records. A patient's right to access to his or her medical records is not without restriction. There is no constitutional property right to one's medical record information. In fact, courts generally have required that the information requested to be disclosed must fulfill a legitimate need for the patient. Generally, such a need has been characterized as that which is necessary to facilitate further health care or to evaluate a legal action. The request for such information must be specific. Courts have upheld denials of requests to inspect medical records where such a request was for no specific purpose and was not narrowed to a type of information.

Some courts have upheld provider denials of patient requests for access to medical information on the grounds that the release of such information might adversely affect the patient's health and well-being. However, courts have upheld denials by providers only in cases where the denial is based on the professional judgment of a physician and where it is properly documented.

Third Party Access. In certain instances, third parties are permitted access to medical information contained in a patient's medical record. The law generally permits medical personnel to have access to a patient's record where there is a legitimate purpose for such access. In addition, a patient may authorize the release of medical information through the execution of a valid consent. Absent a statutory provision to the contrary or a legal guardian contesting such release, a parent of a minor may gain access to the minor's records upon request.

Certain federal laws may permit access to patient medical records by federal agencies without consent by the patient. For example, intermediaries acting on behalf of HHS under the Medicare program may examine medical records in connection with a hospital's annual Medicare audit. Similarly, state agencies that require mandatory reporting of certain patient information, such as birth, death, certain types of procedures (abortions), sexually transmitted diseases or other communicable diseases, child abuse, the prescription of certain drugs that are subject to abuse, and gunshot or other wounds often seen as a result of a violent crime, are statutorily granted access to patient-specific medical information. Finally, state medical disciplinary boards responsible for investigating physician misconduct are typically granted access to patient records through court orders. Some courts have required the removal of patient identifying information absent a special showing of a compelling state interest in the release of the medical information contained in the patient's record.

Conclusion

Legal considerations will continue to be of significant concern to CDMs in a variety of operational situations. While obtaining legal input may be perceived as a cost in the short term, a CDM is likely to experience long-term operational benefits and efficiencies as a result of seeking legal assistance in instances where uncertainty exists.

References

1. *Smith v. Van Gorkom*, 488 A.2d 858 (Del. 1985).

2. *Mills Acquisition Co. v. Macmillan, Inc.*, 559 A. 2d 1261 (Del 1989).

3. *Stearn v. Lucy Webb Hays Sch.*, 381 F. Supp. 1003 (D.D.C. 1974).

4. *Warren v. Wheatly*, 331 S.W.2d 843 (Ark. 1960).

5. *Mahmoodian v. United Hosp. Ctr., Inc.*, 404 S.E.2d 750 (W.Va. 1991); *Stiller v. LaPorte Hosp., Inc.*, 570 N.E.2d 99 (Ind. Ct. App. 1991).

6. *Granetti v. Norwalk Hosp.*, 557 A.2d 1249 (Conn. 1991); *Gates v. Holy Cross Hosp.*, 529 N.E. 2d 1014 (Ill. 1988).

7. *Anne Arundel Gen. Hosp. v. O'Brien*, 432 A.2d 483 (Md. 1981). Contra *Weary v. Baylor Univ. Hosp.*, 360 S.W.2d 895 (Tex. 1962).

8. *Greisman v. Necomb Hosp.*, 192 A.2d 817 (N.J. 1963).

9. *Rosenblit v. Superior Court*, 231 Cal. App.3d 1434 (Ct. App. 1991); *Ascherman v. Saint Francis Memorial Hosp.*, 45 Cal. App. 3d 507 (Ct. App. 1975).

10. AHA Peer Review Immunity Task Force, American Academy of Hospital Attorneys. *Immunity for Peer Review Participants in Hospitals: What is it? Where Does It Come From? How Do You Protect It?* Chicago, Ill.: American Hospital Association, 1989, p. 6.

11. Health Care Quality Improvement Act, 42 U.S.C. §§ 12001 *et seq.*

12. Health care entities include hospitals, medical groups, health maintenance organizations, and other entities that conduct peer review and provide health care services.

13. There is actually some debate as to whether the failure to report a particular adverse action against a physician will result in the immunity not being available for that action. Despite some ambiguity on the issue in the case law, a strict reading of the statute and regulations suggests that the immunity should continue in effect until the Secretary of Health and Human Services notifies the institution and gives it an opportunity to correct alleged deficiencies. Only if noncompliance continues would the immunity be lifted, after publication of the entity's name in the *Federal Register*.

14. Civil Rights Act of 1964, 42 U.S.C. §§ 2000(a) *et seq.*,

15. Hill-Burton Act, 42 U.S.C. §§ 291 *et seq.*

16. *Cook v. Ochsner Found. Hosp.*, 319 F. Supp. 603 (E.D. La. 1970).

17. *Ritter v. Wayne County Gen. Hosp.*, 436 N.W.2d 673 (Mich. Ct. App. 1988).

18. *Arline v. School Bd. of Nassau County*, 107 S. Ct. 1123 (1987).

19. Opinion of the General Counsel, District of Columbia (Oct. 15, 1985).

20. *Simkins v. Moses H. Cone Memorial Hosp.*, 323 F.2d 959 (4th Cir. 1963), *cert. denied*, 376 U.S. 938 (1964).

21. *Eaton v. Grubbs*, 329 F.2d 710 (4th Cir. 1974).

22. N.Y. Pub. Health Law § 2803-c(h).

23. *Lucy Webb Hayes Nat'l Training School v. Geoghegan*, 281 F. Supp. 116 (D.D.C. 1967).

24. 42 U.S.C. § 1395dd.

25. The COBRA designation derives from the fact that the antidumping provisions were part of the Consolidated Omnibus Reconciliation Act.

26. 42 U.S.C. § 1395dd-(a).

27. The definition of emergency medical conditions now encompasses women experiencing contractions. Formerly, the definition of emergency medical condition involved whether the patient was experiencing active labor.

28. 42 U.S.C. § 1395dd-(h).

29. 42 U.S.C. § 1395dd-(b).

30. 42 U.S.C. § 1395dd-(a).

31. 42 U.S.C. § 1395dd-(b)(3).

32. *Stevinson v. Enid Health Sys., Inc.*, 920 F.2d 710 (10th Cir. 1990).

33. 42 U.S.C. § 1395dd-(c)(1).

34. 42 U.S.C. § 1395dd-(c)(1)(A)(ii).

35. 42 U.S.C. § 1395dd-(c)(2).

36. *Sorrells v. Babcock*, 733 F. Supp. 1189 (N.D.Ill. 1990).

37. 42 U.S.C. § 1395DD-(d)(1)(a).

38. 42 U.S.C. § 1395dd-(d)(1)(B).

39. 42 U.S.C. § 1395dd-(d)(1)(c).

40. 42 U.S.C. § 1395dd-(d)(2)(B).

41. 42 U.S.C. § 1395dd-(d)(2)(a).

42. *Schloendorff v. Society of New York Hosp.*, 105 N.E. 92 (N.Y. 1914).

43. *Sanders v. Nouri*, 688 S.W.2d 24 (Mo. App. 1985); *Kahoutek v. Hafner*, 366 N.W.2d 633 (Minn. Ct. App. 1985).

44. *Salgo v. Leland Stamford, Jr. University Board of Trustees*, 317 P.2d 170, 181 (Cal. Ct. App. 1957).

45. *Hook v. Rothstein*, 316 S.E.2d 690 (S.C. Ct. App. 1984).

46. *Paige v. Manuzek*, 471 A.2d 758 (Md. 1984).

47. *Stafford v. Louisiana State Univ.*, 448 So.2d 852 (La. Ct. App. 1984).

48. *Dewes v. Indian Health Serv.*, 504 F. Supp. 203 (D.S.D. 1980).

49. *Karlsbeck v. Westview Clinic*, 375 N.W.2d 861 (Minn. Ct. App. 1985).

50. *Davidson v. Shirley*, 616 F.2d 224 (5th Cir. 1980).

51. *Magana v. Elie*, 439 N.E.2d 1319 (Ill. Ct. App. 1982).

52. *Natanson v. Kline*, 350 P.2d 1093 (Kan. 1960).

53. *Hawaii v. Standard Oil Co.*, 405 U.S. 251 (1972).

54. *In the matter of Kathleen Farrell*, 529 A.2d 494 (N.J. 1987) (refusal of mechanical ventilation upheld on basis of right to privacy); *St. Mary's Hosp. v. Ramsey*, 465 So. 2d 666 (Fla. Ct. App. 1985) (refusal of treatment based on religious grounds upheld).

55. *Farrell* (court recognized common law right to self-determination); *Bouvia v. Superior Court*, 225 Cal. Rptr. 297 (Ct. App. 1986) (discontinuation of nasogastric feeding upheld in part based on public policy codified in California's "Natural Death Act").

56. *Cruzan v. Director*, 110 S. Ct. 2841 (1990).

57. *Crouse Irving Memorial Hospital, Inc. v. Paddock*, 485 N.Y.S.2d 443 (Sup. Ct. 1985); *Application of Winthrop University Hospital*, 490 N.Y.S.2d 996 (Sup. Ct. 1985).

58. *Fosmire v. Nicoleau*, Civ. Act. No. 267 (N.Y. Ct. App. January 18, 1990) (pregnant Jehovah's Witness permitted to refuse a blood transfusion based on religious grounds).

59. *In re Quinlan*, 355 A.2d 647 (N.J. 1976) (incompetent patient's right to self-determination based on constitutional right of privacy).

60. *In re Custody of a Minor*, 379 N.E. 2d 1053 (Mass. 1978).

61. *Md. Family Law Code Ann.* § 5-203b.

62. *In re Eric B.*, 235 Cal. Rptr. 22 (Ct. App. 1987) (Christian Scientist parents ordered to submit their child to periodic medical evaluation, even though the child's cancer was in remission, because of the court's finding that failure to do so would pose an unreasonable risk of harm to the child).

63. *In re Hofbauer*, 393 N.E.2d 1009 (N.Y. 1979).

64. *In re Phillip B.*, 156 Cal. Rrptr. 48 (Ct. App. 1979).

65. *In the interest of E.G.*, 515 N.E.2d 286 (Ill. App. Ct. 1987) (Seventeen year old minor permitted to refuse blood transfusion based on his expressed religious beliefs).

66. *Application of Cicero*, 421 N.Y.S.2d 965 (Sup. Ct. 1979) (court ordered life-sustaining treatment against parents' objections); *Weber v. Stony Brook Hosp.*, 456 N.E.2d 1186 (N.Y. 1983) (court upheld parents' choice of nonsurgical treatment for severely disabled newborn).

67. 42 U.S.C. § 5101.

68. *Barber v. Superior Court*, 147 Cal.App.3d 1006 (Ct. App. 1983).

69. *Roe v. Wade*, 410 U.S. 113 (1973).

70. *Whalen v. Roe*, 429 U.S. 589 (1977).

71. *In re B*, 394 A.2d 419 (Pa. 1978).

72. *Illinois v. Florendo*, 447 N.E.2d 282 (Ill. 1983).

73. M.D. Health Gen. Code § 4-301.

74. *Sklager v. Greater Southeast Community Hosp.*, 625 F. Supp. 991 (D.D.C. 1984).

75. *JCAHO Accreditation Manual*, §§ MR.3 to MR.3.4.

76. *Underlying Principles of Medical Ethics*. Chicago, Ill.: American Medical Association.

77. *Patient's Bill of Rights*. Chicago, Ill.: American Hospital Association.

Mark E. Lutes is an attorney in the Washington, D.C., office of Epstein, Becker & Green, P.C. Neil S. Olderman is an attorney with the Washington, D.C. firm of Green, Stewart & Farber, P.C. Both authors represent a wide range of health care providers and payers.

CHAPTER 12

Issues of Quality

by Marianne D. Kanning, MD,
Charlotte K. Ellingson, ART, and Beth A. Fischer, ART

*I*ssues of quality are not new.[1] In 1917, the American College of Surgeons created the first hospital accreditation standards. One page in length, these standards served as a guide for improving hospital performance and for promoting high-quality care. The standards formed the basis for the first voluntary accreditation program in health care. In 1951, the American College of Surgeons, the American Medical Association, the American Hospital Association, the American College of Physicians, and the Canadian Medical Association banded together to create the Joint Commission on Accreditation of Hospitals. The Joint Commission required that the medical staff review the quality of medical care provided but gave little specific guidance about how this was to be done.

In 1974, a specific standard, "Quality of Professional Services," was developed, stating just how patient care was to be reviewed. Interpretation of this standard evolved into the audit process. A certain number of audits, depending on the number of hospital admissions, were required to be completed by the medical staff. The process was criticized for being too prescriptive and allowing little latitude in interpretation. Creativity in the review of care was stifled. The numbers requirement deteriorated into a numbers game. Any hospital could be sure of "credit" as long as the required number of audits were completed, even though there were absolutely no findings other than "failure to document."

By 1979, the audit process was considered a failure and was abandoned. In place of the Quality of Professional Services standard, a new standard, called "Quality Assurance," was developed. Hospitals became accustomed to playing a numbers game with audits. This continued to play out with the Quality Assurance program. The legend grew, even though it was untrue, that the various hospital departments had only to do a certain number of studies per year to comply with the standard. Medical staffs abandoned all audit efforts and returned to the traditional surgical case review, blood usage review, medical records review, pharmacy and therapeutics review, antibiotics review, and clinical case presentation. These were performed perfunctorily and ineffectively. Because the Joint Commission promised to enforce the quality assurance standard, gradually such quality assurance activities were given "credit." Thus, the legend was perpetuated, even though the only findings were "failure to document" or "variation justified."

As a result, the problem-focused approach to quality assurance evolved. Rather than looking at many aspects of a randomly chosen topic in an effort to discover problems that may or may not have existed, quality assurance started with a known problem or issue in which a problem was suspected. Studies, as a primary means of problem identification, were eliminated. Problems soon surfaced with the problem-focused approach. Most problems identified were administrative in nature or pertained to lack of documentation; few clinical issues surfaced. The medical staff continued to perform its continuous monitors ineffectively. Most problem cases were justified. The approach to quality assurance was modified once again.

In 1984, the requirements for review of patient care became much more specific. The vague "review of medical care" was defined as "meetings to consider the findings from the ongoing monitoring and evaluation of the quality and appropriateness of the care and treatment provided to patients." A new quality assurance section spelled out requirements for the medical staff quality assurance program. An important part of the ongoing monitoring of care was the so-called continuous monitoring activities of the medical staff—as previously mentioned, surgical case review, blood usage review, medical records review, pharmacy and therapeutics review, and antibiotic review (changed to drug usage review in 1986). This monitoring had been done by discrete groups, usually committees, but the findings never before were used in the overall medical staff review of care. In addition to the revised medical staff standards, the entire quality assurance program and all quality assurance units were required:

✦ To have a planned, systematic, and ongoing process to monitor and evaluate patient care.

✦ To collect or screen information about patient care on an ongoing basis.

✦ To periodically evaluate that information for possible problems.

✦ To resolve problems and improve care.

Along with new standards came a tougher survey process. Ineffective review of patient care was assigned as recommendations by the surveyors and most of the recommendations concerning quality assurance became compliance assessment factors. This approach promised to be effective and economical. Data collection was ongoing and reviewed constantly. The flow of information was complex. No longer was it possible to prepare for a JCAHO survey in two months of hard work. It required consistent attention, but also promised improved patient care.

The 1980s were years of dramatic change in the U.S. health care delivery system. There were major reforms in payment mechanisms for hospitals and physicians and the development of more intense provider competition. Perhaps the most far-reaching change was that the country's longstanding priority for quality was reshaped by compelling demands for greater efficiency in the delivery of services and for far more objective evidence of the effectiveness of care.[2]

In the 1990s, however, those who pay for and consume health care expect an objective accounting of the results of care. Organizations that are able to demonstrate that they provide care in a cost-effective and efficient manner are likely to be winners in this new environment. Balance in the relationship between quality and cost must become the new objective in health care. Attention must now be devoted to applying and improving methods for the assessment and improvement of patient care. In this effort, health care managers, governing bodies, and health care practitioners must work together far more closely to evaluate and improve the processes that lead to the efficient delivery of high-quality care—that lead to real value. This must be a cross-organizational initiative that involves conscious effort to overcome traditional but artificial internal barriers. This striking change in public policy and societal expectations occurs at a time when a major reevaluation is already under way within the Joint Commission. There are mounting indications that the steady accretion in the volume of standards results in a blurring of the evaluation focus and, indeed, of performance expectations. It becomes clear that the historical concentration on analysis of capability needs to be supplemented by the monitoring of actual performance.[3]

Those who have followed the Joint Commission standards, particularly the quality assurance standards, for the past few decades will have noticed the evolution of means to assess and improve quality in health care.[4] Implicit peer review was followed by medical audits, and medical audits were followed by ongoing monitoring and evaluation.[5] Today, a new, more positive approach called continuous quality improvement is emerging in health care. This movement is adapting the philosophy and tools that industries have used for years to effectively improve the levels of quality in their products and services. If we can use the tools of continuous quality improvement to achieve greater efficiencies in the delivery of health care services, reduce costs, and improve quality, we will have done much to reassert the private sector's leadership for high-quality health care.

Skilled leaders are critical to set the stage for medical quality management. The health care industry needs visionary leaders with the basic qualities of integrity, trust, and respect for health care providers in their institutions. Experience and observation have suggested that this is lacking in a vast number of health care organizations. Quality management programs fail because of the lack of leadership. Historically, hospital administrations have delegated the quality management function mainly to nurses and occasionally to medical record professionals. It has been the responsibility of these two groups to coordinate quality management functions with the medical staff, hospitalwide ancillary departments, nursing departments, and administration. This is often done piecemeal, without an established process that includes all components of established standards and outside regulatory requirements.

The outcome of this leadership approach is quality management programs varying from nonexistent to exceeding standards in various departments/ services in individual institutions. The variance in quality programs largely depends on the level of understanding, priorities, political barriers, culture, and mentality of CEOs, senior management, and middle management. There is a lack of employee involvement in departmental quality management programs. Often, the manager or a delegated assistant has full responsibility for data collection, action, and follow-up, with little or no staff involvement. A comprehensive and detailed vision of the big picture, with all loops closed, needs to be agreed upon, established, and supported by the CEO and senior and middle management of all departments/services before implementation.

JCAHO reports that failure to meet medical staff standards makes up more than one half of Type I contingencies, while nursing services has a higher compliance. Nurses proudly proclaim that they comply; it is the medical staff that doesn't cooperate. It is our experience and observation that medical staffs with leaders who have the ability to set the stage with a well-defined, comprehensive, and detailed process for defining quality, setting standards, monitoring performance, and determining outcomes will buy into and benefit from the process. The medical staff is often expected to be in compliance with JCAHO standards with little or no direction from hospital administration and quality management program directors. Many hospitals do not have a volunteer or a paid medical director who acts as a liaison between administration and the medical staff to assist in coordination of medical staff requirements.

There needs to be an identified process and systematic approach, with parameters outlining medical staff requirements, standards, and responsibilities to accomplish a true quality management program. Volunteer members of the medical staff are expected, despite busy medical practices, to magically design, implement, monitor, and evaluate quality management programs that include all the key factors of JCAHO requirements. There is a lack of leadership/support from hospital administrations/management to see the big picture of why quality management programs fail or are ineffective. No longer can mediocrity be tolerated...at any level. The attitude "we're no worse than anyone else" or acceptance of thresholds of less than 100 percent must be eliminated. Twenty-first Century leaders must replace old-style managers (see figure on page 187).[6]

The success of the Quality Management Program at St. Francis Regional Medical Center, Shakopee, Minnesota, is credited to the key ingredients of excellent rapport with physicians; ongoing education, including one-to-one teaching; and a well-planned process based on a concurrent, systematic approach that is tried, tested, and true. The process is fair, nonthreatening, and educational. It allows

How to Manage for Continuous Process Improvement[1]

"A manager's primary responsibility to subordinates is to identify and remove or reduce all barriers that could, in any significant way, prevent the individual employee from doing the pest possible job."

DO THIS	NOT THIS
Seek the cause of a problem by examining the process. Accept that 90 percent of all problems are process issues, only 10 percent are human errors.	Assume that "somebody" must have done something wrong, blame them, and discipline appropriately.
Use work teams throughout the organization to study processes and make recommendations for continuous improvement.	Believe that only technical specialists have the knowledge and training to improve processes.
Understand internal supplier-cutomer concepts and the interdependence of all processes.	Allow turf building between and among departments.
Manage to continually improve all processes and reward reductions in variation.	Establish theoretical standards and quotas. Punish for not meeting quotas. Demand productivity beyond capability and capacity of system.
Respect, understand, and accept variability and normal distribution in all processes.	Demand perfection, zero defects, error-free work.
Build trust within the organization by driving out fear.	Allow fear to serve as a control. Do not accept or recognize that fear exists in every organization.
Realize that old paradigms may hinder progress; recognize and accept new paradigms.	Cling to the philosophy that traditional management styles have worked in the past, so why change. "If it ain't broke, don't fix it."
Display an active, visible commitment to continuous process improvement, adjusting personal leadership style as necessary and expecting all managers to join in the change.	Offer lip service to C.P.I. and continue the practice of top-down decision making.
Study and seek to understand the teaching of Dr. W. Edwards Deming, including his Fourteen Obligations of Management.	View Deming as just another theorist, C.P.I. as just another fad.
Understand and use the Shewhart Cycle-Plan, Do, Check, Act—when making a change. Require sound, accurate data upon which to base decisions. Determine real cause(s) before making a change.	Manage by reflex. Use own version of Shewhart-Act on a symptom; Hope the solution works; Pray if it doesn't.
Have a good working knowledge of the problems identification and problem-solving tools—brain-storming, cause-and-effect diagram flowcharts, data collection, Pareto Graph, run charts, control charts, histograms, and normal distribution.	Use gut-level feelings, intuition, and monthly reports to solve a problem.
Welcome messengers.	Shoot messengers.
Maintain high level of understanding the ultimate customers' wants, needs, and expectations.	Assume all is well unless customers complain.

us to work together to maintain and improve the quality of patient care. The JCAHO Ten Step Methodology to quality management is in place hospitalwide[7]:

1. Assign responsibility.
2. Delineate scope of care.
3. Identify important aspects of care.
4. Identify indicators of care.
5. Establish thresholds for evaluation.
6. Collect and organize data.
7. Evaluate care.
8. Take action.
9. Assess action.
10. Report and communicate findings.

This process, along with an annual appraisal/evaluation of departmental monitoring and evaluation activities, is mandatory in every department. The appraisal must include summarization of outcomes of patient care, reporting improvements, policy or practice changes, education or training programs, changes in forms or systems, customer satisfaction, and safety/risk issues.

Our institutional goal is to administer the highest quality of care. The medical staff and administration support an active program to promote high-quality care and to provide for the welfare and safety of patients, employees, medical staff, and visitors. The governing board has delegated the responsibility of monitoring, peer review, and evaluation of this care to the medical staff and administration. In 1985, the decision was made to implement Craddick's Medical Management Analysis approach to quality management. The program has been in place since October of that year.

What are the goals of our Quality Management Program?

✦ To improve quality of care and utilization of hospital resources.

✦ To reduce personal injuries.

✦ To reduce liability risks and claims.

✦ To meet requirements of regulatory agencies.

✦ To provide data on clinical competence for informed medical staff privileging.

✦ To integrate quality improvement philosophies into monitoring and evaluation and all quality management activities.

What are the objectives of the Quality Management Program?

✦ Comprehensive review of all hospitalized patients, using objective criteria that apply to all providers of care on an equal basis.

✦ Timely identification of problems in patient care through concurrent record review and immediate professional attention to adverse events or patterns of care.

✦ Effective and efficient quality and cost control through coordination of all peer review activities, such as utilization management, medical care evaluation, surgical case review, drug usage, and infection control.

✦ Demonstration of objective improvement in the quality of care through problem-directed actions, continuing medical education, and continuous reevaluation for improvement.[8]

Thomas Luth, MD, Quality Management Committee Chairman, notes, "The Quality Management Committee at St. Francis Regional Medical Center plays a key role in the maintenance of high standards of care. Its presence is now accepted, although reluctantly at times, but it does motivate open discussion among members of the medical staff, with action on quality issues. Although sometimes hard to maintain, the educational intent of the process remains the primary goal. Because of this goal, the program continues to function effectively and to succeed in continuous quality improvements as confirmed by our recent JCAHO survey. There has also been a dramatic improvement in chart documentation as a result of ongoing support and education from the Quality Management Committee and a high level of awareness and compliance by the medical staff and other health care providers."

David Willey, MD, Quality Management Committee member and past chairman concurs. "Quality management at St. Francis is intended to be an educational task. The committee has created a system that gathers meaningful data that can translate into action for improved patient care and satisfaction. Quality management indicators have been forcing us to look at outcomes of events for each department and for each physician, and this is done in a most confidential manner. If problems are identified as urgent or with repeated occurrence, the involved persons are informed with an intent of discovery and educating for change. Where action has been necessary from the committee's viewpoint, follow-up changes have occurred without incident. Over the six years the system has been in effect, the medical staff has been on a learning curve of how to make the process meaningful and to justify and trust the result as being, in fact, an opportunity to improve care rather than fear it as judgmental. We have seen the medical staff, as a result of the process, work better together at problem solving. Strategies for improved patient care now also consider consumer/patient satisfaction as a major factor."

What is Medical Management Analysis?

Medical Management Analysis (MMA) is a comprehensive, efficient, effective, and systematic approach to quality management and risk management. As its name implies, MMA is a management system for the objective analysis of medical and other hospital care. At the heart of MMA is the process of occurrence screening, in which all patient care is reviewed (concurrently and retrospectively) against a set of general outcome screening criteria. Adverse patient occurrences (APOs) are identified, confirmed by peers, trended in an automated confidential database, and appropriately followed up. Our software was customized to our institutional needs by a local software company for a very reasonable fee.

What are distinctive elements of MMA that make it "comprehensive, efficient, effective, and systematic?"

Comprehensive: All patient records are screened, not just a sample. The MMA screening criteria identify 80-85 percent of the adverse patient occurrences in the hospital, compared to 30 percent for the best incident reporting programs.

Efficient: Instead of multiple overlapping chart reviews, a single chart screener meets the data collection requirements not only of quality management and risk management, but also of medical staff peer review, infection control, nursing, drug usage, surgical case review, and utilization management for cost control purposes. MMA data are also used as one tool for monitoring performance as part of the credentialing process.

Effective: Serious events are reported immediately to the appropriate department, committee, or individual for prompt follow-up action. All APOs are entered into a confidential, automated database that is used to identify patterns of care and potential problems involving patient care.

Systematic: The medical staff and hospital facilitate timely assessment, follow-up action, problem resolution, monitoring, and documentation of results.

What is an adverse patient occurrence?

Is that just another term for negligence? No. An APO is an untoward patient event that, under optimal conditions, is not a natural consequence of the patient's disease or treatment. The confirmation of an APO does *not* necessarily imply negligence on the part of the provider. APOs include falls, burns, misdiagnoses, surgical mishaps, and unexpected disabilities and death. Studies published in the *New England Journal of Medicine* and other professional journals have documented that, depending on the type of care, 5-20 percent of hospitalized patients will experience APOs. These are not necessarily episodes of negligence. They are events that peers have agreed are *not* what should happen under optimal conditions and reflect what peers want to examine when they monitor the quality of care.

The MMA screening criteria objectively identifies APOs for further assessment. By studying and responding to APO data, hospital departments and peer review committees focus their efforts productively on serious APOs and patterns of suboptimal care. If an APO is confirmed, the reviewer determines whether the standard of care was met. This decision can be made only by a peer. One of three options are assigned:

✦ **The standard of care was met (+).** This means that the APO was confirmed and trended, but, in the opinion of the reviewer, there was no associated negligence on the part of any person or the institution. The majority of APOs are not associated with any breach of care standards.

✦ **The standard of care was questionable (+/-).** This means that the reviewer might have managed the situation differently, but there was no clear breach in the standard of care. In these cases, the reviewer may also elect to refer the chart to a committee or a department for further evaluation. This is especially appropriate in smaller hospitals where physicians must review some charts outside their specialties.

In some hospitals, all cases with questionable care must have a further review by either the department chief or the quality management committee. In some cases, the involved practitioner is invited or required to participate in the discussion for educational purposes.

✦ **The standard of care was not met (-).** In these instances, the reviewer decides that most prudent physicians, given the same set of circumstances, would not have behaved in a similar fashion, and, thus, the practitioner under review breached the standard of care. In many hospitals, particularly smaller ones, this decision may be too difficult for a physician reviewer to make alone. The reviewer may elect to refer this record to the department chairman or a small ad hoc group for additional evaluation. APOs determined to be the result of failing to meet the standard of care may have potential liability. The quality management coordinator should notify risk management, if this has not already been done.

The peer reviewers also assign a severity code to every APO:

0 = no disability
1 = minor temporary
2 = minor permanent
3 = major temporary
4 = major permanent
5 = potential major or major continuing
6 = death
7 = noninjury hospital occurrence

Record Documentation Deficiencies (RDDs) are also assigned. These are defined as any missing, untimely, illegible, inappropriate, conflicting, or altered documentation in the medical record that could adversely affect quality of care or create a malpractice risk. RDDs are not assigned a severity code.

When peer reviewers need clarification/rationale of patient care, health care providers receive letters of inquiry. A two-week response time is allowed before

191

peer reviewers assign a standard of care. Health care providers are informed of any questionable (+/-) or negative (-) standard of care assigned to their cases.

What are the MMA Screening Criteria?

There are three basic phases to the criteria:

Monitoring and Problem Identification

✦ Using the medical staff-approved criteria/indicators, screeners review patient charts within 24 hours of admission during regular working days and at regular intervals thereafter. Concurrent reviews are performed on nursing units; retrospective reviews are performed within two weeks of discharge.

✦ Variations from the criteria/indicators are recorded and described briefly on an abstract form.

✦ Screeners also review charts for utilization management, risk management, infection control, nursing, drug usage, and surgical case review. In addition, the Quality Management Department coordinates other data-gathering efforts. In many facilities, there are often several people from various departments/services screening charts for all of these functions.

Assessment

✦ The quality management coordinator reviews all variations from the criteria and determines if they will require secondary review by a peer.

✦ Variations are then referred to a secondary (peer) reviewer who reviews the abstract along with the chart to determine:

—Does the variation constitute an APO?

—If it does, was the standard of care met?

✦ Serious APOs are referred for immediate response, usually to the appropriate department chief. Charts that fall out through the screening process, reflecting nursing variances, are referred to nurse managers for review. Each nursing service's charts are cross-reviewed and assigned a standard of care. Medical staff peer reviewers assess nursing assignments following review through the regular process. Nurse managers bring results to their specific departments, where managers and staff discuss the care issue and take action. Occurrences attributed to ancillary departments/services are assessed through regular medical staff peer review, and results are referred to ancillary department managers for action and follow-up with department staff. Another mechanism used to identify potential quality care issues is through a transmittal process. Transmittals provide a pathway for written notification of a potential APO or other quality concerns that may not be identified in the specific screens. These are forwarded to the Quality Management Department and routed through the regular peer review process.

✦ All APOs are trended in an automated confidential database and reported monthly by department at the specific clinical department meetings. Patterns that may require further study are periodically analyzed in the form of focus studies.

Follow-up Action, Problem Resolution, and Documentation

✦ As appropriate, on a monthly basis, MMA trending data and individual trends are reviewed by the Quality Management Committee, where the results of quality management review and evaluation studies are assessed and recommendations made to the appropriate clinical departments. These recommendations are referred to the chiefs of the departments, who, in turn, choose one or two department members to review and assess. If they feel there is a trend, they discuss this with the involved physicians and make their recommendations. If the individual physician agrees, these recommendations go to the Executive Committee. If the individual physician disagrees, he or she has the option of having the trend sheet discussed at the departmental meeting (anonymous or not), and the recommendations are made to the Executive Committee. The Executive Committee evaluates and implements corrective actions. If a further recommendation and/or plan of action is needed, the problem is referred to administration and the governing board.

✦ The Quality Management Committee reports quality management activities to the specific clinical departments, the Executive Committee, administration, and the governing board.

✦ Through ongoing monitoring, MMA identifies and documents the effectiveness of actions taken.

✦ MMA also provides ongoing monitoring and objective documentation for physician credentialing and other required medical staff peer review functions.[9]

According to the quality management team at Saint Francis Regional Medical Center, "Successful identification of problems and positive problem solving has occurred in the past six years at SFRMC because of the willingness and support of our physicians. They are compliant and objective in their peer review responsibilities. We view the Quality Management Program at St. Francis Regional Medical Center as an educational, fair, nonthreatening approach of working together to maintain and improve the quality of patient care. It is a way to help each other keep current with criteria and documentation requirements of governing agencies and hospital accreditation organizations."

St. Francis Regional Medical Center ranked in the top 3 percent of hospitals nationwide by the JCAHO in August 1990, receiving no Type I recommendations in its on-site survey in June 1990. Along with the accreditation came an official letter of commendation from the President of the Joint Commission, Dennis O'Leary, MD, FACPE, stating, "St. Francis Regional Medical Center received an overall accreditation grid score of 90 or above (out of a possible 100), which places your organization among the most effective accredited organizations."

During the JCAHO on-site review, the survey team recognized St. Francis Regional Medical Center to be unique and to excel beyond other institutions surveyed. This was demonstrated by total commitment to quality through a team effort of the governing board, medical staff, administration, medical director, nursing, and support staff. The survey team was particularly impressed with the unusually high level of physician participation. Their dedication to the quality management process was recognizable throughout the hospital and emphasized the great opportunity St. Francis Regional Medical Center has to move ahead in a competitive medical environment with a "team who has it together." Because of this, the quality management team is responding to requests from other hospitals for consultative services. The quality management team shares its experience/ expertise through on-site evaluation assessments, providing insight into the facility's "gaps and/or overlaps" in existing quality management programs.

CQI, TQM Come to St. Francis Regional Medical Center

St. Francis Regional Medical Center is moving ahead with continuous quality improvement. It is imperative that the CQI process be built on the strengths of a successful traditional quality management program. Traditional quality management plus continuous quality improvement equals total quality management. Senior management cannot depend on consultants or simply purchase one of the many expensive TQM packages flooding the market. It should take the responsibility to assess the strengths and weaknesses that are already in place and to customize the CQI process, focusing on strategy, cultural change, and statistical and quantitative measures/methods. Senior management needs to be careful not to mandate participative management before it empowers the staff.

The communication/environment process at Saint Francis Regional Medical Center is a process that is being integrated into every department's current traditional Quality Management Program not only to identify problems but also to help change systems to avoid problems in the future. This process focuses on communication and environment. It teaches staff members the value of overcoming the fear to communicate honestly and openly with one another and of taking responsibility for their actions. It is designed to provide insight into the staff's perception of departmental goals. The procedure is based entirely on staff consensus. An inhouse facilitator meets initially with department staff to identify areas of concern. When the identifying and prioritizing process is completed, the results are submitted, along with appropriate recommendations/resolutions, to the department director and to other appropriate administrative persons. A follow-up meeting is scheduled at which supervisory personnel respond to the proposed resolutions in terms of agreement, disagreement, or tabling.

Follow-up meetings with time lines are scheduled for all agreed to and tabled items. Monitoring of resolutions is ongoing between staff and administrative personnel and should be included in regular staff meetings. The process is repeated every six months. This process is the basis for empowering the staff to communicate intradepartmentally, thus setting the stage for interdepartmental communication, as most of the systems problems are found in "the cracks" where departments/systems interface. When interdepartmental problems/ systems failures are identified through this process, appropriate quality improvement teams are established for problem solving. Ideas leading to profit and problem resolution come from employees closest to the problems, those in the trenches.

Celebrating success is the most powerful tool to enhance employee enthusiasm. We have a motto at SFRMC: "Our Spirit is Contagious." All employees, medical staff members, and governing board members were given a top-quality tee shirt imprinted with this motto and St. Francis Regional Medical Center's logo. It is important to recognize employees for their ideas and efforts—even kinder-gartners will "kill" for a gold star.

Traditional quality management/good medicine/doing the right things plus continuous quality improvement/common sense/having the right things in the right place at the right time equals total quality management.

References

1. *The New Quality Assurance: Third Generation.* Irving, Tex.: Dallas-Fort Worth Hospital Council, 1985.

2. *Anesthesia and Obstetrical Quality Indicators: Beta Phase Training Manual & Software User's Guide.* Oakbrook Terrace, Ill.: Joint Commission on Accreditation of Healthcare Organizations, 1990.

3. *The Joint Commission's Agenda for Change: Stimulating Continual Quality Improvement in the Quality of Care, 1990 Indicator Driven Monitoring Systems,* Chapter Two. Oakbrook Terrace, Ill.: Joint Commission on Accreditation of Healthcare Organizations, Feb. 1990.

4. *The Transition from QA to CQI: An Introduction to Quality Improvement in Health,* Chapter One. Oakbrook Terrace, Ill.: Joint Commission on Accreditation of Healthcare Organizations, 1991.

5. *Transitions from QA to CQI Using CQI. Approaches to Monitor Evaluate and Improve Quality.* Oakbrook Terrace, Ill.: Joint Commission on Accreditation of Healthcare Organizations, 1991.

6. *How to Manage for Continuous Process Improvement.* Gerald Donley, Certified Consultant, Menominee, Wis., 1991.

7. *JCAHO Ten-Step Methodology.* Oakbrook Terrace, Ill.: Joint Commission on Accreditation of Healthcare Organizations, 1986

8. Medical Management Analysis, Joyce Craddick, MD, Auburn, Calif., 1983.

9. Spath, P. "QA Professionals Must Begin Continuous QI Process." *Hospital Peer Review,* June, 1991, pp. 87-9.

Marianne D. Kanning, MD, is Medical Director; Charlotte K. Ellingson, ART, is Quality Management Program Manager; and Beth A. Fischer, ART, is Quality Management Program Specialist, St. Francis Regional Medical Center, Shakopee, Minnesota.

CHAPTER 13

Overseeing Cost–Effectiveness in the Provision of Medical Care

by Alan H. Rosenstein, MD, MBA

By the end of 1991, health care spending will total over 700 billion dollars, accounting for almost 12 percent of the U.S. Gross National Product. At the same time that health care spending continues to rise, the health care dollar is becoming an increasingly limited resource. Government, the number one purchaser of health care services (accounting for 40 percent of health care spending), is concerned about diminishing funds to support Medicare and Medicaid programs. Industry, the second major purchaser of health care services (accounting for 37 percent of health care spending, with average employee health care premiums exceeding $3,000 per year) is concerned about the erosion of corporate profits and its ability to provide comprehensive health care services to employees. With this growing concern over health care spending, health care payers are beginning to scrutinize the health care system, making providers more responsible for the entire process and outcome of health care delivery. As part of their efforts to control health care costs, health care payers enacted significant changes in utilization controls and reimbursement restrictions in a direct attempt to shift more of the financial risk to the health care provider. With the hospital as the primary focus, the first series of changes included direct utilization controls and reimbursement limitations that have had a profound effect on hospital-related services. In the second series of changes, payers have extended their focus to include both outpatient and physician-related services, with payments to providers eventually being linked to effectiveness of care. With one payer eye on appropriateness and necessity for health care services and another on efficiency, effectiveness, and outcome of health care interventions, providers are being held more accountable for services rendered. As hospitals and managed care organizations face increasing pressure to manage patients effectively, department chairman and other physicians in leadership positions must play a more active role in managing their departments' performance and efficiency.

Previous chapters have dealt with establishing the roles and responsibilities of clinical department chiefs as effective department managers. Here, we extend their departmental responsibilities to include a focus on cost-efficiency. While high-quality care remains the number one priority, department chiefs must also concentrate on managing departmental activities in terms of physician performance and the cost-effectiveness of care. A model designed to assist the department chief in this endeavor is presented in the following pages.

Background/Financial Risk

Beginning in the early 1980s when government-sponsored TEFRA legislation set the precedent for change from the customary fee-for-service system, health care providers have had to readjust their format for health care delivery. Payments by diagnosis, payments per diem, capitation, and other forms of discounted contractual care have switched the financial risk from the health care payer to the health care provider. As managed care continues to invade the medical marketplace, the fee-for-service patient will soon become a protected species, accounting for a diminishing percentage of inpatient care.

As illustrated in table 1, page 199, hospitals may assume a significant economic liability for patient admissions, lengths of stay, and services provided. For Medicare admissions, the emphasis should focus on ensuring the clinical necessity of the admission, reducing the length of stay, and limiting services provided. For Medicaid and other per-diem admissions, the emphasis is on ensuring the necessity of admission, justifying the necessity of continued length of stay, and limiting services provided. For patients covered by capitation, the emphasis is to avoid the admission, reduce the length of stay, and limit inpatient services by encouraging more outpatient care. For other discounted services, the financial risks and economic incentives vary with the degree of contractual discount. Note at the bottom of table 1 that reimbursement incentives for physician-related services may be contrary to the hospital's reimbursement priorities, as, for the most part, physicians continue to be reimbursed on a fee-for-service basis for inpatient care. The only time hospital and physician economic incentives are aligned is when they both are reimbursed under a fee-for-service or capitation system. As a direct result of these changes, many hospitals have had a difficult time making ends meet.

While high-quality care remains the number one priority, we cannot ignore the economic impact of services provided. With more than 50 percent of hospitals operating at a loss, financial stability becomes a significant concern, and hospital survival may ultimately be at stake. The physician, as the ultimate controller of health care utilization, must become more conscious about the economic as well as quality impact of services rendered.

Hospital Reaction—High-Quality, Cost-Efficient Care

The hospital's primary concern is to provide high-quality, cost-effective care to its patient population. I have taken the liberty of dividing this priority into three separate but interrelated strategies (table 2, page 200).

Table 1. Economic Incentives by Payer Mix

Economic Incentive	Admission	LOS	Resources Used
For Hospitals			
Full charge[1]	+	+	+
Discounted charges[2]	+?	+?	+?
Payment per case[3]	+?	-	-
Payment per diem[4]	+?	+??	-
Capitation[5]	-	-	-
For Physicians			
Full charge[1]	+	+	+
Discounted charges[6]	+	+	+
Payment per case[7]	+?	+	+
Payment per diem[8]	+	+?	+?
Capitation[9]	-	-	-

+ = desirable/increase, - = undesirable/decrease

1. Reimbursed for services provided. For physicians, fee-for-service.
2. Preferred-provider organizations (PPOs): Reimbursed on percentage of charges; the question is whether discounted reimbursement is enough to cover costs.
3. Prospective payment (DRGs): Fixed payment, with emphasis to do less; the question is that it is subject to "admission approval."
4. Medicaid: Paid by the day, with the emphasis to do less; the questions are that it is subject to "admission approval" and payment may be only for "medically necessary" days.
5. Payment per enrollee (HMOs): Money is paid "up front," with incentive to do less.
6. (PPOs) Same incentives as for fee-for-service.
7. Medicare (DRGs): Physicians are reimbursed for services provided; the question is that Medicare may deny payment for unnecessary services.
8. Medicaid: Physicians are reimbursed for services provided; the question is that Medicaid may deny payment for unnecessary services.
9. Physicians may be on fee-for-service reimbursement, with hospital on capitation.

The first and foremost strategy is to ensure high-quality care. Under the guidance of traditional quality assurance and quality indicators, infection surveillance and infection control, continuous quality improvement, total quality management, or whatever you choose to call it, hospitals must focus on the content and process of what they do in an effort to monitor and improve the quality of care. Reductions in complications, adverse events, or other unwanted outcomes have a desirable effect on both quality and costs of medical care. This strategy has obviously been the main responsibility of the department chair and doesn't require further elaboration here.

Table 2. Hospital Reaction

Maintain High-Quality Care

+ Reduce adverse outcomes
+ Reduce unwanted events
+ Reduce unwanted complications
+ Maintain infection control

Utilization Management

+ Appropriateness of admission/ procedure
+ Continued stay review
+ Appropriate level of care
+ Retrospective case-mix review

Resource Management

+ Reduce unnecessary services
+ Avoid duplication of services
+ Substitute less costly services
+ Emphasize cost-effective care

The second strategy deals with effective utilization management through utilization review. Under this category, attention is given to monitoring health care services for appropriateness and necessity of medical care, expediency and timeliness of medical care, and treatment of patients at the most appropriate level of care. The process is divided into three stages (figure 1, page 201). Preadmission review is designed to ensure the appropriateness of the admission based on established severity-of-illness and intensity-of-service medical criteria. The second component focuses on admission and concurrent review. This process is designed to monitor the progress of the hospitalized patient as the proposed treatment plan unfolds and to assess the necessity for ongoing continued acute hospital stay. The third component focuses on retrospective review and case-mix analysis, looking for trends or variances that should be targeted for further review.

The third strategy deals with efficient resource management and identification of priorities for improving the cost-efficiency of care.

When we focus on reducing health care costs in the inpatient setting, we look at two different areas. The first is length of stay. With average inpatient costs of $625 per day, reducing the length of hospital stay by even one day can provide a significant cost-savings benefit. Since the introduction of Medicare's prospective payment system in the early 1980s, coupled with significant advancements in outpatient health care technology, lengths of stay in the hospital have dropped more than 10 percent. Considering that most of the fat has already been trimmed, I'm somewhat doubtful about achieving significant reductions in lengths of stay in the near future. The problem that we face now is that, despite reductions in length of stay and total inpatient days, the consumption of ancillary resources has remained the same or even increased. Their use has just been packed into a shorter time. If more than 50 percent of the patient's bill comes from ancillary charges dictated by the physician's pen, programs designed to monitor and improve ancillary resource utilization will be the next major step in reducing health care costs. The goal of a resource management program is to identify how and where the resources are being utilized and, through data analysis, information sharing, and physician input and participation, to develop appropriate alternatives designed to improve the overall efficiency of care. Once alternatives have

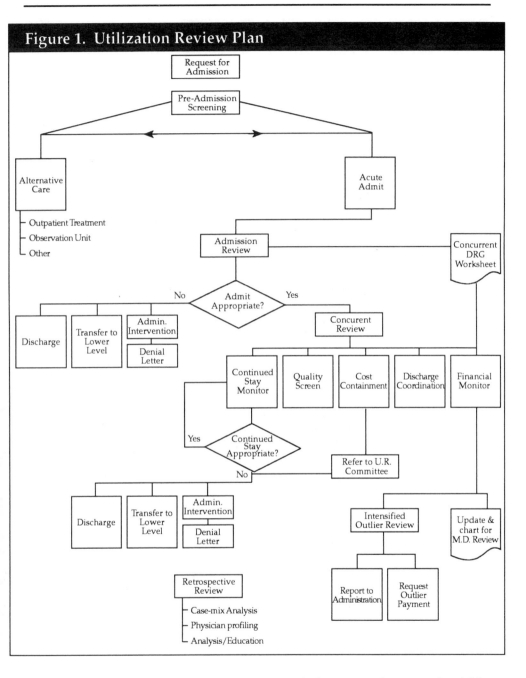

Figure 1. Utilization Review Plan

been developed, a comprehensive program of physician education should be used as the instrument for change. The remainder of this section will be devoted to the development of the resource management model.

One of the first considerations is to decide on what to study and how to set priorities. While this step depends on the institution's individual needs, the concepts

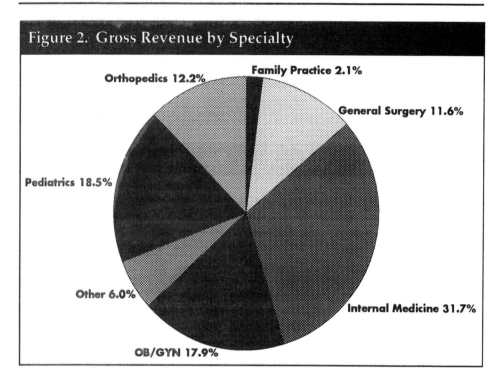

Figure 2. Gross Revenue by Specialty

presented below can be used as a beginning framework.

One of the first things to consider is how your department fits within the hospital as a whole. Individual departments, as well as individual physicians, may be aware internally of how they are performing but have little knowledge of how they perform in comparison to their peers. In an attempt to bridge this "information void," individual departments can compare their activities on the basis of any number of factors considered important for analysis. Figure 2, above, gives an example of one institution's analysis comparing clinical departments on the basis of gross revenues from patient charges. This type of information becomes important in setting institutional priorities for physician recruitment or joint venturing, or for consideration of equitable budgetary allotments for departmental acquisitions, future purchases of new equipment or other capital expenditures. Most important of all, it allows individual departments to see how they are doing in comparison to other units.

An early step in the resource management process is to identify priorities for study. Priorities may be selected on the basis of high volume, high cost, high risk, or other parameters. Table 3, page 204, gives an example of the top 25 hospital diagnoses, based on patient volume. Gross revenues are based on charges, while net revenue indicates the amount of reimbursement actually received, a function of payer mix. Operating costs are the total costs (fixed and variable) incurred for services provided. Profit and loss states the difference between net revenues and operating costs. Note the number of negative profit margins in this area. Figure 3, page 206, illustrates this point more dramatically by plotting the top 10 diagnoses in a more graphic fashion. Table 4, page 205, lists the top 25 least profitable diagnoses by degree of loss. Good thing this hospital had only one case of botulism. Also note that five of the top 25 diagnoses were in the area of cardiac services. We'll return to this point later.

This same type of analysis can be performed by individual departments. Table 5, page 207, for instance, gives a breakout of inpatient surgical services with analysis of revenues based on payer mix. The same type of analysis can be performed for same-day surgery or other outpatient services.

Data analysis of this kind can help the hospital target areas of concern for further study. Each hospital should set its priorities on the basis of its needs. The following section describes selected case studies that illustrate the process in more detail. The first case study will focus on a medical diagnosis using congestive heart failure. The second study will focus on a surgical diagnosis using major joint procedures. As will become obvious during the discussion, different diagnoses will focus on different points for analysis.

Case Study 1: Medicine—Congestive Heart Failure

Using the process outlined above, we can apply the model to analysis of individual department activity. Table 6, page 208, gives a list of the top 25 inpatient diagnoses for the Department of Medicine. Referring back to tables 3 and 4, pages 204 and 205, we note that cardiac-related services represented a significant portion of the overall hospital's inpatient activity, which, unfortunately, also placed the hospital at significant financial risk. With this concern in mind, we proceeded to perform a more in-depth analysis of cardiac services, using congestive heart failure for our initial study.

In the study year, there were 171 cases of congestive heart failure admitted to the hospital. Table 7, page 209, gives an overview of all 171 cases on an case-by-case basis. To focus on where the money was actually being spent, each case is broken out into specific resource centers. Gross revenues again indicate the total charges for that patient, net revenues the amount of payment received, operating costs the total cost of services rendered, and profit and loss the difference between net revenues and total costs. Variable costs or marginal costs are the additional costs of providing that specific procedure, and contribution margin represents the difference between net revenue and variable costs. Note that the analysis dissects gross revenues into charges allocated to specific resource centers. The bottom of the table gives a summary of charges for all 171 cases.

For a medical diagnosis, most of the charges will accrue as room charges, laboratory charges, respiratory therapy charges, pharmacy charges, and charges for other ancillary services. Room charges can be described as fixed charges (daily room rates) to cover room, board, and nursing services, while ancillary charges represent a variable charge based on what the physician orders in the way of

Table 3. Top 25 Diagnoses by Patient Volume

Rank	ICD-9 Code	Principal Diagnosis	Cases	Length of Stay	Gross Revenue	Net Revenue	Operating Cost	Profit/(Loss)	Patient Days
1	V3000	Single Liveborn-in	2810	3.32	7,548,660	5,647,153	5,589,033	58,120	9,343
2	V5810	Maintenance Chem	252	2.46	1,055,205	874,040	807,495	66,545	620
3	65421	Prev C-Sect NOS-	241	3.34	1,047,546	809,712	975,767	(166,055)	805
4	65000	Normal Delivery	200	1.85	446,444	362,150	414,921	(52,771)	370
5	65981	Complic Labor NE	174	2.02	433,117	372,050	389,797	(17,747)	352
6	64403	Thrt Prem Labor-A	173	4.89	651,890	680,085	625,858	54,227	846
7	49391	Asthma w Status As	157	3.16	723,585	445,858	555,430	(109,572)	497
8	42800	Congestive Heart F	149	6.63	1,511,475	965,173	1,300,064	(334,891)	987
9	66411	Del w 2 Deg Lacera	149	2.06	363,656	318,212	328,712	(10,500)	307
10	64421	Early Onset Deliver	143	4.59	884,739	766,866	819,709	(52,843)	656
11	65631	Fetal Distress-Deliv	140	2.99	560,944	443,959	525,525	(81,566)	419
12	48600	Pneumonia, Organis	137	5.46	1,040,974	757,342	837,715	(80,373)	748
13	66331	Cord Entabgle NEC	120	1.91	284,882	247,136	309,438	(62,302)	230
14	65821	Prolong Rupt Memb	115	4.27	646,897	610,382	580,526	29,856	491
15	66401	Del w 1 Deg Lacera	115	1.85	267,352	217,025	246,306	(29,281)	213
16	65341	Fetopelv Dispropor	104	4.21	608,457	471,163	576,912	(105,749)	437
17	66311	Cord around neck-	95	2.05	246,710	196,265	225,975	(29,710)	194
18	65221	Breech Presentat-D	93	4.28	517,614	414,951	500,404	(85,453)	398
19	55890	Noninf Gastroenteri	90	2.62	222,115	199,220	195,753	3,467	236
20	43600	CVA	85	6.11	559,262	495,639	481,817	13,822	519
21	78020	Syncope and Collap	83	2.78	352,415	250,409	314,763	(64,354)	230
22	60000	Hyperplasia of Pros	82	3.14	337,004	322,049	333,090	(11,041)	257
23	65811	Prem Rupt Membra	80	2.41	243,865	212,974	222,972	(9,998)	193
24	78650	Chest Pain NOS	80	1.98	298,528	172,453	270,250	(97,797)	158
25	72210	Lumbar Disc Displa	79	5.67	457,614	411,800	421,822	(10,022)	448
		Total	5,946	3.36	21,310,949	16,664,066	17,850,053	(1,185,987)	19,954

Table 4. Top 25 Least Profitable Diagnoses by Gross Revenue

Rank	ICD-9 Code	Principal Diagnosis	Cases	Length of Stay	Gross Revenue	Net Revenue	Operating Cost	Profit/ (Loss)	Patient Days
1	42800	Congestive Heart Fail	149	6.63	1,511,475	965,173	1,300,064	(334,891)	987
2	510	Botulism	1	99.00	248,206	67,100	208,636	(141,536)	99
3	65421	Prev C-Sect NOS-Deliv	241	3.34	1,047,546	809,712	1,007,267	(197,555)	805
4	41110	Intermed Coronary Syn	58	3.72	385,066	224,495	345,053	(120,558)	216
5	55700	AC Vasc Insuff Intest	2	33.30	174,205	50,355	147,867	(97,512)	67
6	49280	Emphysema NEC	11	12.68	250,295	100,502	198,129	(97,627)	140
7	15320	Mal Neo Descend Col	7	11.96	199,172	64,268	159,351	(95,083)	84
8	73500	Hallux Valgus	9	2.40	34,555	36,823	129,074	(92,251)	22
9	78650	Chest Pain NOS	80	1.98	298,528	172,453	270,250	(97,797)	158
10	49391	Asthma w Status Asth	157	3.16	723,585	445,858	555,430	(109,572)	497
11	65341	Fetopelv Dispropor-Deli	104	4.21	608,457	471,163	576,912	(105,749)	437
12	41070	Subendocardial Infarct	31	7.11	377,890	242,179	333,269	(91,090)	221
13	21810	Intramural Leiomyoma	40	3.74	206,978	144,439	222,503	(78,064)	149
14	V5840	Postsurg Aftercare NEC	29	4.78	290,886	177,243	255,635	(78,392)	139
15	16230	Mal Neo Upp Lobe Lu	20	9.09	317,378	199,138	278,612	(79,474)	182
16	48210	Pseudomonal Pneum	4	18.00	196,638	84,953	158,345	(73,392)	72
17	20500	Acute Myeloid Leukem	8	14.85	250,106	117,252	190,371	(73,119)	119
18	75800	Down's Syndrome	1	31.50	100,270	21,350	87,597	(66,247)	32
19	65221	Breech Presentat-Deliv	93	4.28	517,614	414,951	500,404	(85,453)	398
20	3843	Pseudomonas Septicem	1	108.90	256,298	158,622	229,472	(70,850)	109
21	15050	Mal Neo Lower 3rd Eso	3	13.80	113,666	33,755	96,679	(69,924)	41
22	65631	Fetal Distress-Delivered	140	2.99	560,944	443,959	525,525	(81,566)	419
23	41090	Myocardial Infarct NOS	17	6.19	196,679	101,735	165,913	(64,178)	105
24	15400	Mal Neo Rectosigm J	5	15.12	173,954	82,991	145,219	(62,228)	76
25	76830	Fetal Distress Dur Lab	1	41.40	118,603	28,060	85,104	(57,044)	41
		Total	1,212	4.63	9,158,994	5,658,529	8,172,682	(2,514,153)	5,612

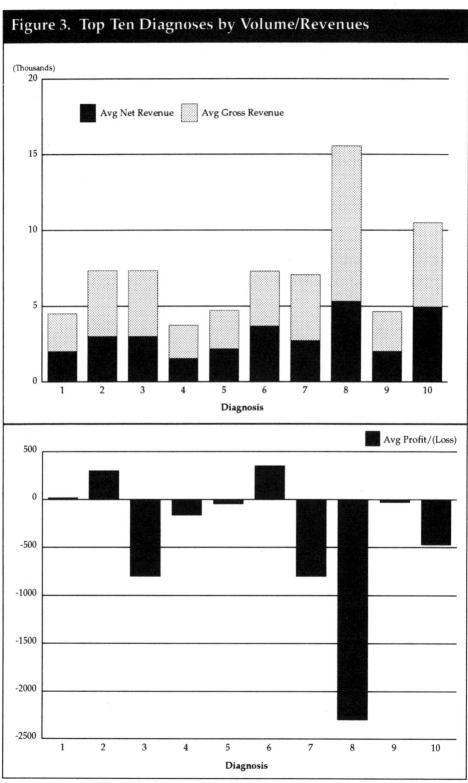

Figure 3. Top Ten Diagnoses by Volume/Revenues

Table 5A. Top 25 Diagnoses by Volume for General Surgery

Rank	ICD-9 Code	Principal Diagnosis	Cases	Patient Days	Average LOS	Gross Revenue	Net Revenue
1	57410	Cholelith W	50	229	4.6	518,111	248,867
2	54090	Acute Appen	32	118	3.7	241,614	131,241
3	44020	Atheroscler	25	361	14.4	730,565	392,054
4	17440	Mal Neo Bre	21	77	3.7	169,073	119,719
5	17480	Malign Neop	19	63	3.3	139,874	71,067
6	23300	CA in Situ Br	17	51	3.0	115,015	55,992
7	54000	AC Append W	17	167	9.8	317,169	153,641
8	78900	Abdominal P	15	57	3.8	80,893	46,880
9	15410	Malignant N	15	193	12.9	366,814	245,596
10	56081	Intestinal A	14	244	17.4	445,259	301,402
11	57400	Cholelith W	13	112	8.6	219,697	99,149
12	43310	Carotid Art	12	78	6.5	212,643	97,923
13	15330	Mal Neo Sig	12	176	14.7	330,843	203,432
14	56090	Intestinal O	11	68	6.2	87,235	60,122
15	17490	Malign Neop	11	38	3.5	80,635	44,464
16	56211	Diverticulit	10	145	14.5	244,569	115,002
17	22600	Benign Neop	9	30	3.3	65,976	26,119
18	44422	Lower Extre	8	149	18.6	348,076	154,196
19	19300	Malign Neop	7	38	5.4	77,745	16,394
20	55010	Unilat Ing H	7	29	4.1	59,111	18,251
21	45520	Int Hemorrho	6	29	4.8	45,724	26,172
22	15360	Malign Neo As	6	123	20.5	244,145	137,779
23	44140	Abdom Aorti	5	84	16.8	262,928	101,300
24	57420	Cholelithias	5	25	5.0	61,496	26,345
25	16230	Mal Neo Upp	5	87	17.4	197,235	58,588
		Subtotal	**352**	**2,771**		**5,662,445**	**2,951,695**
		Avg. per Case			**7.9**	**16,086**	**8,385**

Table 5B. Analysis of Payer Mix on Gross Revenue

Rank	Medicare Revenue	Medicaid Revenue	Commercial Revenue	Neg Cont Revenue	HMO Revenue	Self-Pay Revenue
1	97,800	53,469	43,879	156,607	146,356	0
2	1,519	2,860	58,994	111,715	33,394	8,132
3	423,222	129,509	40,932	0	121,902	0
4	43,442	2,661	77,967	6,541	18,462	0
5	31,399	3,441	14,945	52,873	12,230	0
6	6,294	139	24,110	43,833	20,639	0
7	0	74,134	34,214	162,503	17,654	8,664
8	10,503	0	15,857	14,189	18,829	0
9	140,620	28,849	71,694	0	110,651	0
10	126,931	0	95,449	53,461	154,418	0
11	57,733	54,167	14,390	8,753	45,092	14,562
12	13,151	32,668	22,273	12,214	112,337	0
13	137,712	0	33,695	6,431	138,005	0
14	8,055	0	8,815	20,771	34,594	0
15	18,671	4,806	5,084	13,745	18,329	0
16	91,131	0	18,904	51,295	68,239	0
17	0	0	3,853	28,043	24,080	0
18	113,361	5,288	17,413	17,509	174,505	0
19	2,205	3,269	1,203	11,688	11,166	23,214
20	24,196	10,592	0	10,848	0	0
21	4,108	2,875	14,904	0	8,837	0
22	147,067	20,809	8,975	13,514	33,780	0
23	129,554	0	14,328	16,188	87,858	0
24	10,409	0	0	33,297	7,790	0
25	30,069	24,483	340	20,609	101,734	0
Subtotal	**1,669,152**	**454,019**	**642,218**	**866,627**	**1,520,881**	**54,572**

Table 6. Top 25 Diagnoses by Volume Internal Medicine

Rank	ICD-9 Code	Principal Diagnosis	Cases	Patient Days	Ave LOS	Gross Revenue	Net Revenue
1	V5810	Maintenance Chem	439	1189	2.7	2,563,149	1,541,970
2	42800	Congestive Heart	249	1223	4.9	2,549,416	1,138,142
3	48600	Pneumonia, Organi	163	761	4.7	1,304,698	676,536
4	78650	Chest Pain NOS	143	234	1.6	512,683	204,722
5	42731	Atrial Fibrillation	133	315	2.4	685,656	280,847
6	41110	Intermed Coronary	122	252	2.1	542,286	228,290
7	27650	Hypovolemia	111	318	2.9	432,424	259,618
8	43600	CVA	109	445	4.1	692,046	342,208
9	43490	Cerebr Artery Occ	104	511	4.9	737,497	448,522
10	78020	Syncope and Colla	96	129	1.3	223,171	108,095
11	57810	Melena	90	260	2.9	482,307	184,505
12	78900	Abdominal Pain	86	143	1.7	189,198	86,476
13	46600	Acute Bronchitis	85	214	2.5	381,930	168,890
14	28262	HB-S Disease with C	84	119	1.4	129,143	96,629
15	13630	Pneumocystosis	84	467	5.6	877,531	555,861
16	59900	Urin Tract Infecti	84	251	3.0	339,490	157,604
17	55890	Noninf Gastroente	82	137	1.7	184,744	84,714
18	41390	Angina Pectoris NE	81	100	1.2	163,522	69,967
19	43590	Trans Cereb Ische	81	113	1.4	126,192	69,064
20	40291	Hyperten Heart Di	79	184	2.3	249,925	146,190
21	49391	Asthma w Status A	76	210	2.8	441,310	143,241
22	41011	Ami Anterior Wall	76	224	2.9	555,645	207,525
23	53140	Chr Stomach Ulc	75	205	2.7	442,530	201,105
24	57700	Acute Pancreatitis	74	208	2.8	296,975	122,434
25	68260	Cellulitis of Leg	74	174	2.4	176,334	100,946
		Subtotal	**2,880**	**8386**		**15,279,802**	**7,624,101**
		Average per Case			**2.9**	**5,305**	**2,647**

Table 7. Case Summary DRG 127, Congestive Heart Failure

Case	LOS	Age	Gross Revenue[1]	Net Revenue[2]	Operating Costs[3]	Profit/ Loss[4]	Variable Costs[5]	Contribution Margin[6]
1	3	56	6,671	2,460	4,436	(1,976)	1,932	528
2	7	54	12,370	4,270	8,531	(4,261)	3,776	494
3	24	89	23,510	19,600	15,522	4,158	6,562	12,118
4	40	71	81,904	32,880	56,506	(23,706)	25,635	7,166
5	9	67	16,354	7,435	11,493	(4,058)	5,065	2,369
6	10	68	12,153	5,971	6,737	(776)	1,682	4,288
7	11	57	13,580	9,020	7,276	1,744	1,883	7,137
8	5	85	13,150	4,100	7,898	(3,798)	3,441	659

Case	Pharmacy Charges	Respiratory Therapy/ Pulmonary Function Charges	X-ray Charges	Lab Charges	ECG Charges	Room Charges	Other Ancillary Charges
1	506	95	269	1,325	410	3,850	216
2	530	493	373	2,579	733	7,400	262
3	1,881	3,144	688	3,300	174	12,220	2,103
4	7,434	1,742	713	6,353	133	52,740	12,789
5	1,287	394	460	1,471	485	11,025	1,232
6	1,174	1,612	73	2,456	485	5,750	603
7	1,426	1,581	217	3,578	64	6,050	664
8	659	1,959	401	2,291	625	6,125	946

Total Cases	Avg LOS	Avg Age	Avg Gross Revenue[1]	Avg Net Revenue[2]	Avg Operating Costs[3]	Avg Profit/ Loss[4]	Avg Variable Costs[5]	Avg Contribution Margin[6]
171	7.03	73	11,810	6,575	7,835	(1,260)	3,393	3,182

Total Case	Avg Pharmacy Charges	Average Respiratory Therapy/ Pulmonary Function Charges	Avg X-ray Charges	Avg Lab Charges	Avg ECG Charges	Avg Room Charges	Avg Other Charges
171	830	994	294	1,974	317	6,598	803

1. Based on hospital charges.
2. Based on anticipated payments (adjusted for payer mix).
3. Based on total (allocated) costs.
4. Derived from Net Revenue–Operating Costs.
5. The actual additional costs of services provided.
6. Derived from Net Revenue–Variable Costs.

diagnostic and therapeutic services. Note in this case that ancillary charges account for almost 45 percent of the average patient's bill. Table 8, below, summarizes, in a similar fashion, average physician-specific data for total cases with this diagnosis.

Having accumulated all these data, the real work is about to begin. After the data have been aggregated, they are presented to the department chairman for analysis. Trends in resource consumption, as well as variances in the patterns of care, can be identified. With the department chairman taking the lead, the next step was to present these data to the individual department members at the next department meeting. All department members were forwarded a cover letter explaining that we would be discussing physician trends in congestive heart failure at the next meeting. As part of the package, we included a basic definition of certain economic terms and a confidential "disidentified" physician summary profile report where individual physicians would recognize where they stood in relation to their peers. At this meeting, we discussed the economic concerns that most hospitals were experiencing in the treatment of congestive heart failure. We

Table 8. Physician Summary for DRG 127, Congestive Heart Failure

Physician ID#	Total Cases	Avg LOS	Avg Pharmacy Charge	Avg Respiratory Charge	Avg X-ray Charge	Avg Lab Charge	Avg ECG Charge
A	4	8.8	1,711	1,233	415	2,539	423
B	2	7.0	1,126	480	344	1,969	109
C	1	11.0	2,440	3,107	352	5,812	599
D	3	7.0	552	693	288	1,818	717
E	6	6.2	645	472	292	2,264	367
F	4	6.5	758	1,031	297	2,360	464
G	5	4.6	524	739	278	1,409	250
H	1	5.0	370	25	112	1,685	144

Physician ID#	Avg Gross Revenue	Avg Net Revenue	Avg Operating Costs	Profit/ (Loss)	Avg Variable Costs	Avg Contribution Margin
A	18,024	10,274	14,767	(4,493)	6,247	4,027
B	14,484	9,503	11,706	(2,203)	5,192	4,311
C	28,852	9,229	26,323	(17,094)	12,001	(2,772)
D	9,953	7,509	7,975	(465)	2,878	4,631
E	11,717	5,906	10,100	(4,194)	4,447	1,459
F	11,888	7,059	9,617	(2,588)	4,072	2,987
G	7,683	3,910	6,771	(2,861)	2,825	1,085
H	6,752	6,267	5,194	1,074	1,728	4,540

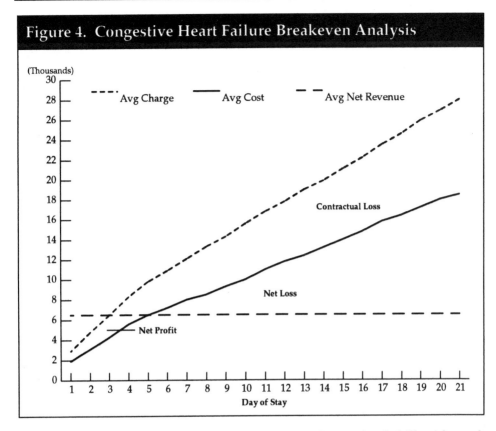

Figure 4. Congestive Heart Failure Breakeven Analysis

began the discussion by presenting a representative patient's bill with total charges for the hospital stay summarized according to room rates and ancillary services described previously.

After presenting this summary, we provided a graphic description of a break-even analysis summary of the 171 cases of heart failure (figure 4, above). The top curve represents the cumulative summary of total daily patient charges and the lower curve represents the cumulative summary of actual costs of care. The horizontal straight line across represents the average reimbursement received from all payer classes. After day two of hospitalization, there is a contractual loss representing the negative balance between charges and net reimbursement. This is a paper loss. However, we run into a real net loss after day five, where costs begin to exceed net reimbursement. The net profit section in this graph appears to be very small, and it leaves little opportunity to generate profit. So how can you maximize the net profit portion? First, reduce the length of stay. Obviously, this is economically advantageous for patients reimbursed under a fixed case payment, as in Medicare, or for patients covered by capitation, but it may not be economically advantageous for patients covered under a fee-for-service or per-diem reimbursement. The second strategy is to lower the cost line by reducing the amount of services consumed. Lowering the costs of services through this process will be economically beneficial for all cases covered under per diagnosis, per diem, or capitation

211

arrangements. This makes a strong case for efficient resource management.

We can begin by analyzing each resource center in an attempt to uncover any possible trends that may be amenable to improvement through the substitution of more cost-effective alternatives. The first section we studied was laboratory services. We noticed that there were occasions where several individual tests would be ordered that could have been ordered more effectively through specific test panels. Recognizing that most of the physicians were still relatively unaware of specific laboratory charges and that we could improve effectiveness in laboratory ordering by encouraging panel selection rather than individual testing, part of the education process included a discussion of laboratory utilization trends as well as distribution of a panel-price list of laboratory charges. Other issues discussed were indications, timing, and effectiveness of laboratory testing as a possible explanation for the large degree of variance in physician ordering patterns in this area.

Next we looked at pharmacy and respiratory services to see if we could improve efficiencies in these areas. Appropriate utilization of cardiac drugs and drug levels, and appropriate utilization of oxygen therapy and saturation monitoring were also important topics for discussion.

One area that we wanted to pay particular attention to was utilization of special diagnostic tests and procedures for cardiac diagnoses. LDH isoenzymes, blood gases, echocardiograms, stress tests, and thallium scans were analyzed as part of a focus study designed to monitor indications and appropriateness of these procedures. Table 9, page 213, presents an example of such an analysis, with charge and cost data applied to these tests. Given that most of the patients in this group were Medicare, avoiding those tests that were not clinically necessary or could have been performed safely on an outpatient basis would provide a significant savings by eliminating essentially nonreimbursed additional costs. Results were reported in the Fall 1991 issue of *Hospitals and Health Services Administration*.

Case Study 2: Orthopedics—Total Joint Procedures

The second case study is an example of resource consumption in a surgical diagnosis—orthopedics and total joint procedures. Tables 10 and 11, page 214 and 215, summarize hospital and physician activities for 211 cases performed in the study year. Unlike the medical diagnosis in which resource consumption was spread relatively uniformly across ancillary services, in a surgical diagnosis the predominant charges fall into the surgical cost center. Table 12, page 216, breaks out the surgical cost center by physician for DRG 209, total hip procedures. The cost center lists charges for surgery based on charge rates per minute, charges for anesthesia and recovery room, central supply charges, and charges for prosthesis. It is the latter that drew our attention. The range for total hip prosthesis varied from $2,350 for standard hardware to $6,000 for a custom prosthesis, including delivery charges and customized nuts and bolts not currently in stock (table 13, page 216). We'll come back to this point later.

Table 9. Special Study—Diagnostic Tests, Congestive Heart Failure

Case	Lab Charge	LDH Iso-enzymes Charge	LDH Iso-enzymes Cost	Arterial Charge	Arterial Cost	ECG Charge	Echo-cardiogram Charge
A	580	0	0	0	0	350	0
B	887	130	90	170	63	133	0
C	2,013	259	180	0	0	985	346
D	854	65	45	0	0	196	0
E	180	65	45	0	0	127	0
F	746	65	45	0	0	692	346
G	1,419	194	135	0	0	825	346
H	879	130	90	0	0	69	0

Case	Echo-cardiogram Cost	Stress Test Charge	Stress Test Cost	Nuclear Medicine Charge	Thallium Scan Charge	Thallium Scan Cost
A	0	219	118	563	564	390
B	0	0	0	0	0	0
C	187	0	0	365	0	0
D	0	0	0	0	0	0
E	0	0	0	0	0	0
F	187	219	118	563	563	390
G	187	219	118	563	563	390
H	0	0	0	0	0	0

As with the Department of Medicine, we shared the data with the department chief and decided to present this information at the next Department of Orthopedics meeting. Prior to the meeting, each member of the department received a cover letter explaining the purpose of the meeting and defining common economic terms, along with a confidential personal physician profile (table 14, page 217). We began the meeting by discussing how the data were tabulated and used the break-even analysis chart as the basis for discussion (figure 5, page 218). The top curve represents cumulative total patient charges, the lower curve cumulative costs of care, and the horizontal straight line the average reimbursement received, considering all patient classes. Note the relative high costs of care in the first two days. After day two, we head into a contractual loss as the difference grows between charges and net reimbursement, but we do not get into a net loss until day 10. In this case, the net profit area is much larger. Again, there are two primary strategies involved to improve this net profit portion.

Table 10. Diagnosis-Related Group (DRG) Summary Averages, 1987 (Before Study)

DRG No.*	Patients	Avg Length of Stay, days	Avg Age, years	Gross Revenue	Charge/Patient ($)							
					Room	Pharmacy	Laboratory	Surgery	Physical Therapy	Central Services	X-Ray	Other Ancillary Charges
209	129	10.56	66	17,756	5,878	1,036	733	7,381	633	1,158	267	670
210	48	11.71	71	16,302	6,762	1,340	1,492	3,186	586	1,085	798	1,053
211	15	8.93	35	11,022	4,906	973	397	2,953	379	795	372	247
212	19	4.68	9	7,421	2,693	539	263	2,985	89	319	279	254
Total/Average	**211**	**10.18**	**60**	**16,016**	**5,723**	**1,056**	**839**	**5,716**	**556**	**1,040**	**396**	**690**

*DRGs 209 through 212 refer to Major Joint Procedures.

Table 11. Physician Summary Averages

Attending Physician	Patients	Avg Length of Stay, days	Avg Age, years	Gross Revenue	Room	Pharmacy	Laboratory	Surgery	Physical Therapy	Central Services	X-Ray	Other Ancillary Charges
1	2	9.00	70	17,444	4,924	807	950	7,337	618	1,076	218	1,514
2	15	8.87	59	15,881	5,042	1,157	896	6,170	545	1,000	487	584
3	2	6.00	31	6,256	3,299	395	84	2,187	0	245	0	46
4	10	10.80	69	17,416	6,153	1,397	886	6,342	599	1,176	255	608
5	6	10.00	77	15,451	5,909	991	1,337	4,168	574	842	774	856
6	51	10.27	64	17,310	5,652	990	771	7,151	610	1,196	288	652
7	14	9.21	59	12,964	5,155	846	615	4,085	497	819	436	511
8	9	16.44	66	22,693	9,251	1,635	1,224	5,924	1,109	1,506	789	1,255
9	15	10.73	62	19,050	6,261	1,357	1,072	7,106	519	1,739	299	697
10	1	6.00	78	9,135	3,300	161	414	3,091	336	552	810	471
11	28	9.29	57	14,297	5,111	860	587	5,456	516	937	287	543
12	14	6.86	15	11,292	4,039	750	388	4,908	210	498	305	194
13	12	9.50	62	14,312	5,284	972	802	4,754	480	836	522	662
14	3	14.33	68	20,267	7,937	1,063	1,785	6,223	637	1,152	593	877
15	11	11.18	62	16,227	6,150	1,148	719	5,186	505	894	474	1,151
16	7	13.57	83	19,779	8,316	1,628	1,959	3,167	775	1,231	906	1,797
17	8	11.13	62	13,903	6,075	1,277	1,007	3,483	607	514	382	558
18	1	12.00	74	19,411	7,425	916	1,629	5,479	588	1,933	367	1,074
19	1	11.00	80	15,728	5,775	481	590	7,199	511	832	0	340
20	1	5.00	42	9,184	3,015	505	486	4,294	231	301	173	179
Total/Average	**211**	**10.18**	**60**	**16,016**	**5,723**	**1,056**	**839**	**5,716**	**556**	**1,040**	**396**	**690**

Charge/Patient ($)

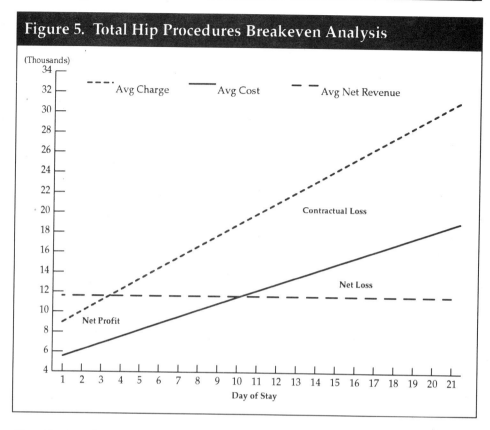

Figure 5. Total Hip Procedures Breakeven Analysis

Considering that most patients requiring total hip surgery are in the Medicare category, with the hospital reimbursed on a fixed payment per diagnosis basis, it would be desirable to reduce the length of stay as much as clinically possible. It's a lot easier to accomplish this in the orthopedic case, for two basic reasons. First, when you're dealing with an average length of stay of 10 days rather than three to five days, there is a lot of potential for movement. Second, in orthopedic cases, the latter days of hospitalization are dedicated more to rehabilitation, and these services can be provided at a lower level of care, such as a skilled nursing unit or rehabilitation facility.

The second strategy is to reduce overall resource consumption. As before, we looked into all the individual resource centers. In the laboratory, we suggested using a hemogram rather than a CBC, a type & screen instead of a type & cross when clinically appropriate, and more standardized laboratory monitoring of anticoagulation therapy. In the pharmacy center, we looked at utilization of pre- and postoperative utilization of antibiotics, analgesia, and I.V. fluids. But the biggest impacts were made in the room cost center and the surgical cost center, as discussed below.

When we presented this information to department members, it became quite apparent that there was a large variance in lengths of stay among physicians and that definite improvements could be made. Recognizing the economic impact length of stay had on total costs of care, the orthopedists agreed that earlier transfer to a skilled nursing unit was indeed appropriate. This proposal was aided by the fact that we have an in-hospital skilled nursing floor. One of the orthopedists suggested that, during the preoperative office consultation, they should discuss with the patient and his or her family that the patient will be spending three to five days in the hospital, followed by another five days in the skilled nursing unit. The patient and family would thus be prepared for the transfer, making the final disposition a lot smoother than trying to wait until the fifth day of hospitalization to begin efforts to transfer the patient to a lower level of care.

Next we discussed the surgical cost center, with a special focus on orthopedic hardware. During the meeting, we distributed a price list of all the different appliances listed on the menu. This was an eight-page document listing over 80 different pieces of hardware. The idea was to substantially reduce the number of pieces held in inventory and encourage use of standard stock items. As one orthopedist put it, why should he use a $6,000 prosthesis if the result would be no different than with a $3,000 one.

The orthopedic case study was the first study we conducted at the hospital. Table 15, page 220, shows the results of the pre- and posteducation period, as reported in the February 1991 issue of the *Western Journal of Medicine*. Overall there was a 10-15 percent reduction in charges, reflective of improvement in the cost-efficiency of care.

Other Case Studies

Several other case studies have been conducted, focusing on other departments and diagnoses as well as on resource consumption through the eyes of the ancillary department.

In the pharmacy, we are in the process of tightening up the formulary and trying to reduce the amount of medications provided at discharge. Specific drug evaluation studies of appropriateness, efficacy, and cost-effectiveness are being conducted in the areas of antibiotic therapy and the use of H_2 blockers. Pharmacy and the departments of medicine, pediatrics, and surgery have combined efforts to present educational rounds promoting effective utilization of antibiotics for the treatment of various types of pneumonia and to recommend appropriate antibiotic utilization in the pre-, peri- and postoperative surgical patient. Similar studies are underway to promote appropriate utilization of respiratory services, laboratory services, and other special procedures, as discussed earlier.

Educational efforts must include a combined effort between ancillary departments and the medical staff. In the era of managed care and reimbursement limitations, ancillary departments must shift their focus from trying to maximize

Table 15. Orthopedic DRG Financial Trend Analysis of an Inlier Population,[1] 1987 and 1988

Population and Services	Hospital Charge 1987	Hospital Charge 1988[2]	% Change
Total Population			
Patients	164	187	14.0
Average length of stay, days	10.1	8.7	-13.9
Average age, years	64	70	
Average charge per patient, $			
Total gross revenue	16,107	15,145	-6.0
Pharmacy	1,051	937	-10.8
Surgery	5,771	5,926	2.7
Laboratory	985	868	-12.9
Physical therapy	564	521	-7.6
Central service	1,027	856	-16.7
X-ray	398	408	2.5
DRG 209, Major Joint Procedure			
Patients	117	116	-0.9
Average length of stay, days	10	8.5	-15.0
Average age, years	66	67	
Average charge per patient, $			
Total gross revenue	17,188	16,513	-3.9
Pharmacy	958	956	-0.2
Surgery	7,377	7,725	4.7
Laboratory	835	711	-14.9
Physical therapy	602	559	-7.1
Central service	1,140	896	-21.4
X-ray	247	242	-2.0
DRG 210, Hip/Femur[3]			
Patients	30	37	23.3
Average length of stay, days	10.5	9.4	-10.5
Average age, years	72	82	
Average charge per patient, $			
Total gross revenue	13,721	13,972	1.8
Pharmacy	963	1,012	5.1
Surgery	2,775	2,929	5.5
Laboratory	1,283	1,339	4.4
Physical therapy	507	506	-0.2
Central service	756	869	14.9
X-ray	744	712	-4.3
DRG 211, Hip/Femur[4]			
Patients	13	29	123.1
Average length of stay, days	10.6	8.7	-17.9
Average age, years	54	78	
Average charge per patient, $			
Total gross revenue	12,254	12,275	0.2
Pharmacy	873	857	-1.8
Surgery	3,001	3,069	2.3
Laboratory	520	924	77.7
Physical therapy	596	462	-22.5
Central service	560	755	34.8
X-ray	535	668	24.9
DRG 212, Hip/Femur[5]			
Patients	4	5	25.0
Average length of stay, days	8.5	8	-5.9
Average age, years	11	8	
Average charge per patient, $			
Total gross revenue	9,600	10,066	4.9
Pharmacy	597	501	-16.1
Surgery	2,655	3,258	22.7
Laboratory	427	446	4.4
Physical therapy	189	168	-11.1
Central service	360	511	41.9
X-ray	356	367	59.3

1. Inlier population is defined as those patients with a length of stay +/-1 standard deviation from the average.
2. Charges are adjusted for price increases between 1987 and 1988.
3. Hip and femur procedures except major joint procedures, in patients 18 years and older, with complications or comorbidity.
4. Hip and femur procedures except major joint procedures, in patients 18 years and older, without complications or comorbidity.
5. Hip and femur procedures except major joint procedures, in patients under 18 years.

departmental revenues to trying manage their departments more effectively by promoting cost-effective utilization of both manpower and resources to benefit the institution as a whole.

Physician Education

The crucial component in providing cost-efficient care lies in the hands of the ordering physician, and this is where the department chairman can play a pivotal role. Physician leadership is vital in any process that requires physician motivation for change. Improvements can be gained from a program that includes information sharing, physician input and discussion, and development of positive alternatives for change. Implementation occurs through the process of physician education, discussion, monitoring, feedback, and control.

The information sharing phase is probably the best place to begin. The autonomous nature of medical practice tends to lead physicians to practice in an information void. The physician may be familiar with his or her own practice style and maybe those of partners but is relatively unaware of how his or her practice patterns compare with those of peers. The information sharing phase is designed to expose the physician to other practice styles to see how he or she compares in the treatment of like conditions.

In going through the information sharing stage, there are several important points to consider before you begin. First is the absolute assurance that the information is to be kept confidential. Second is to present the information in a positive manner. With the threat of everybody looking over the physician's shoulder, it should be made clear that the purpose of gathering such information is not to weed out the bad apple, but for everyone to improve the overall process of care by sharing like experiences. Physicians are basically good people, and they really want to do what's best for their patients. Exposing the physician to peer group performance activities helps establish peer group supported standards for care, and most physicians would like to practice in line with the norm. In our experience, when we have provided physicians with their individual performance profiles, the reaction has not been skepticism, but rather genuine enthusiasm and a desire to get even more information so that they analyze the data even further.

The department chief should take an active role in organizing collected data to the best advantage for the department's needs. The data should be utilized to identify trends or variances in care that may be amenable to improvement. Improvements can be gained by presenting the data to physician users and encouraging their input and suggestions, which lead to the development of specific alternatives designed to improve the process of care. With departmental approval, alternatives are implemented and supported through physician education, and the results are monitored, with the process being revised as needed.

The physician education process provides the vital link for success. Just as important as physician input and participation on the front side is the need for continued reinforcement on the backside. Our experience has shown that educational efforts tend to have a very short half-life and that, in order to continue to produce positive results, the educational efforts must continue on an ongoing basis. This ongoing education can be conducted through monthly department meetings or newsletters, bulletin boards, floor cards, or "post-its," but the best results are obtained if reminders exist at the point of contact. The ideal reminder is a real-time, physician-interactive computer, where certain order entries elicit computer-generated, on-screen prompts that provide the physician with selected additional bits of information at the time of computer access. If you're lucky enough to have such a system, use it to its maximum advantage.

When we look at significant variations in physician patterns of care, the information sharing and education process should be geared to improve the overall spectrum of care. There may be some occasions where the general physician education programs will have to be supported by more individualized efforts when clinically appropriate. When this occurs, the department chief must assume a leadership role.

For institutions with active residency teaching programs, special efforts should be made to include the housestaff as part of the above-mentioned process. If members of the housestaff write most of the orders, you have a wonderful opportunity to educate a captive audience that is still relatively flexible and amenable to change. It still amazes me that that there is still relatively little education at the medical school level on the medical economics of health care delivery. In our institution, we begin a comprehensive medical economics seminar in July to correspond with the new crop of entering interns and residents. The first series of lectures provides an overview of the current health care system. The second series of lectures devotes itself to the impact of health care changes on the hospital sector, which includes discussions on utilization review and managed care. The third series of lectures deals with the choices to be considered by residents contemplating entrance into the real world practice of medicine and the advantages and disadvantages of different practice alternatives. After this structured series of lectures, we begin an ongoing program of selected case studies where residents and staff discuss topics on cost-effective, high-quality care.

A few final suggestions in the physician education arena are in order. First, when we talk about economic incentives being different for different payer classes, we certainly don't mean that physicians should treat patients differently based on their insurance coverage. All physicians should recognize the economic ramifications of what they do and try to treat all patients as effectively and efficiently as possible. Second, the information presented should, whenever possible, be discussed in a positive, constructive manner. Third, the priorities of high-quality care should always be reaffirmed. Fourth, the importance of physician-to-physician interaction should be recognized. The role of education and motivation for change should come from physician leadership and not from administration or finance.

Physician Motivation: Incentives for Change

While the clinical department chief recognizes the importance of providing cost-effective care, the practicing physician, immersed in the intricacies of day-to-day medical practice, may not be as sympathetic to this issue. Preoccupied with concerns about meeting patient's needs and providing high-quality care in the face of an ever-increasing load of paperwork and other administrative burdens, the clinician may exhibit a significant degree of resistance to change. On one side, we note a passive type of resistance that may simply be attributed to a sense of inertia. "I've been doing things this way for 20-odd years now. I don't understand why I have to change." On the other side, we encounter a more aggressive stance from physicians reacting to increasing bureaucratic interference that they feel compromises their ability to provide necessary care. Most physicians recognize that things aren't quite the same as they used to be, but the degree of adaptability and flexibility tends to be related to number of years in practice and physician age. Physicians who have been in practice more than 35 years tend to "roll with the flow" as they recognize that they'll only be in practice for a few more years. It's a little easier to acquiesce than it is to resist the changes that are being forced upon them. Physicians just entering practice are also more accommodating to change, as they have grown up with the concepts of financial risk, managed care, and the looming threat of limited health care resources. Physicians in their early 40s tend to be the hardest nut to crack, as they've been at it for 15 or 20 years and have grown up under the incentives of the traditional fee-for-service reimbursement system. With these differences in mind, let us consider in more detail potential obstacles and incentives and the pros and cons of motivating changes in physician behavior (table 16, page 224).

The first real concern we must address is the perceived impact on quality. Throughout medical school and residency training, physicians have traditionally been taught to use all the resources at their disposal, to leave no stone unturned in an effort to make a firm diagnosis. We have all "searched for zebras" and that extremely rare diagnosis. Under this "quality equals quantity" philosophy, asking physicians to be more judicious about the use of resources is tantamount to treason. But should we expend significant resources for only minimal incremental gains in diagnostic confidence? If we spend $500 and reach a diagnostic confidence level of 95 percent, is it appropriate to spend an additional $500 to increase our diagnostic confidence level to 96 percent? Given the increasing constraints on the health care dollar, maybe we should not. It's not a matter of "quality equals quantity"; it's more a matter of "quality equals efficiency."

Next is the issue of malpractice. Physicians feel obligated to do additional testing or procedures in fear of potential retrospective malpractice allegations, and until there is a significant revision of the legal standards in this area, this situation will continue. There are two responses customarily utilized in an effort to avoid this malpractice. The first is ordering additional tests and procedures to make sure you've covered all the bases. This response is fraught with its own difficulties. Every time you order an additional test or procedure, you are

Table 16. Pros and Cons of Resource Management

Cons:	Pros:
Physician inertia	Hospital survival?
Impact on quality?	Financial Incentives
	Direct-profit sharing?
Malpractice concerns	Indirect-money available?
Economics vs. science	Quality = Efficiency
	"Continuous improvement"
Bad apple approach	
	Internal vs. external control
Economic credentialing	
	Hospital-physician collaboration
Top-heavy administration	contracting joint ventures
	Philosophical imperative
	Hospital loyalty
	Resource management vs. rationing
	Guidelines/indicators/protocols

responsible for follow up and interpretation, and this may end up in a never-ending battle of chasing abnormal results. We must also respect the caveat of "physician do no harm." It has been well documented that exposing patients to additional procedures increases the likelihood of unwanted events. The second response is good chart documentation. Most of the problems arise when the physician knows why and what he or she wants to do, but fails to document his or her thought processes appropriately in the chart. Removal of ambiguities and documentation of patient discussions about treatment alternatives with prescriptions for appropriate follow-up care are the best ammunition for preventing malpractice events.

Next is the issue of economics versus science. We frequently hear concerns about the difficulties of trying to measure a subjective behavioral science by objective economic measures. While it is true that medicine is more of a qualitative science, most patients still fall into regularly identifiable patterns that lend themselves to quantitative measurements.

On the issue of economic credentialing and the concern about hospitals using information to weed out the bad apples, our objective is to use the information in a more aggregate format, moving the entire department to a higher level of achievement. This is consistent more with the goals of continuous quality improvement and total quality management than with singling out individuals in a critical manner.

There is also the issue of trying to reduce costs by reducing the ranks of top-heavy administration. The point is that everybody has to work together and do their parts in an effort to reach a mutual goal. Administration must streamline operations and personnel, secure advantageous purchasing and contracting arrangements, and pursue other cost-containment measures. Ancillary department managers must change their focus from maximizing departmental revenues for the department's good and concentrate on maximizing efficiencies in labor and resource utilization for the good of the institution as a whole. Physicians must raise their level of consciousness about the costs of services provided and strive for more judicious, appropriate, and effective utilization of costly resources.

On the positive side of the picture, we deal with institutional loyalties and institutional survival. Physicians may threaten that they can always pack up and move their services to the hospital across the street, but that is a rather naive perception. In this era of hospital closures, mergers, and consolidations, there may not be a hospital across the street for them to move into. Also, physicians are creatures of habit. They develop very comfortable working relationships with a hospital and rely on it as a familiar workplace. Once a physician leaves a hospital, his or her referral patterns will be disrupted and all those other built-in conveniences, largely taken for granted, are no longer around. Besides, with all hospitals being placed more or less in the same predicament, who's to say the situation across the street is any better than the situation currently at hand?

Financial incentives are probably the strongest motivator of physician behavior. While it is illegal to pay physicians directly for being efficient utilizers, there are several other ways in which physicians can be rewarded for more efficient behaviors. First is the idea of a withholding pool. If the hospital and physician groups participate in certain managed care programs and share in a risk pool, money left over at the end of the year can be distributed to physician members. A second possibility is to tie department improvements and additions to performance efficiency. If there is a limited amount of funds available in the hospital capital budget for department improvements or equipment purchases, allocating dollars according to departmental efficiency may be the most equitable way to distribute the funds. Another way to get physician leaders interested in taking a stronger role in these activities is to assign these activities as part of their departmental responsibilities and pay them accordingly. Nothing works better than paid positions with designated responsibilities. Of course, each institution must decide on the best alternative to follow.

Now we're ready to face the issue of the external them versus the internal us. As mentioned previously, external payers have a very strong financial interest in everything that we do and are spending a lot of time and effort monitoring the process and outcome of care in an effort to make providers more accountable for services rendered. With estimates that 20-30 percent of services provided may not be clinically warranted, appropriateness, necessity, justification and outcome are the new terms being used as the payers look at quality and efficiency of services provided. From the Health Care Financing Administration and the Health Care Quality Improvement Act, to the Joint Commission on Accreditation of Healthcare Organizations and its Agenda for Change, to insurance companies and entrepreneurial utilization review companies, each organization has its own agenda for gathering data in an effort to analyze and criticize what we do. On the surface, the intention is to improve the overall process of care, but the real intention is to measure one provider against the next in an effort to isolate more efficient care givers for the purpose of selective contracting. Some states, such as Pennsylvania, go so far as to publish doctor and hospital batting averages for selected diagnoses. Each organization wants to make you accountable to its own system of data analysis. I feel it is better and more appropriate for us to measure what we do and try to improve ourselves internally, rather than succumbing to external agencies who seem to have their own individual sets of criteria, indicators, or guidelines.

Finally, we must emphasize the importance of hospital-physician collaboration. In today's era of managed care and selective contracting, hospitals and physicians must begin to work together with the goal of providing high-quality, efficient medical care. The system can no longer afford the multitude of problems generated from an adversarial relationship between these two parties. What is needed is increasing cooperation and mutual trust in the formation of mutually beneficial joint ventures and other collaborative efforts designed to improve the efficiency and effectiveness of health care delivery.

The Future

In developing responsibilities for clinical department chiefs, we must also keep an eye on future trends in health care and design their responsibilities accordingly. There appears to be no end in sight for substantial reductions in health care spending. As money becomes more and more limited, we will see a greater focus on selective contracting and attempts to limit resource allocations, with payments being tied to appropriateness, efficiency, and outcome of health care services. Given the multiplicity of customers involved in the health care product, it is important for physician leaders such as clinical department chiefs to play a strong leadership role in reinforcing the need for physicians to be sensitive to the concerns of health care customers. Payers and insurers are primarily concerned about reducing their health care budgets and will continue to try to reduce costs by shifting financial risks to health care providers. Health care providers will have to learn how to manage financial risk in order to maintain financial viability and provide alternatives that lead to more effective and efficient operations. Patients, as the innocent bystanders, will be more concerned about access to care and services covered than actual out-of-pocket costs. It is up to the health care provider to meet patient demands by providing more appropriate allocation of scarce health care resources. Payers, insurers, patients, and providers must all work together to improve the system. Physician leaders must strive to maintain internal control of a system plagued by increasing external constraints.

Alan H. Rosenstein, MD, MBA, is Director of Medical Resource Management, California Pacific Medical Center, San Francisco, California.

EPILOGUE

✦

I am assuming that you have taken or are contemplating taking that plunge into the mysterious waters of medical management. And I am also assuming that, in preparation for that plunge, you aquired this book about medical management, hoping that it would be your life preserver and keep you afloat until you could become proficient in the many life-saving strokes needed in the swirling waters of medical management.

Each of the chapters of this book has been written, reviewed, and edited by members of the American College of Physician Executives who are very actively engaged in some form of medical management. The subjects involve specific directions for aquiring the skills needed to begin the handling of basic problems you may encounter in medical management. Each chapter is, in itself, a mini-lifesaver. Of course, how you handle each of these "life-savers" will depend upon you and the circumstances that you encounter when you need the skills.

Review and application of the many helpful basics found in this volume will be as necessary as review and practice of any life-saving technique. If, after review and practice, there is a need for more help, you will find that not only will the authors be willing to respond to your call of, "help, I'm over my head," but also other experienced members of the College will rush to your aid if they hear your call. Just make the request.

A final word of warning. This treatise is intended to get you started in this administrative ocean. If used correctly, it can keep you afloat. But please be aware that, just as in all other endeavors, there are the unseen dangers. You should be able to survive these dangers and gain even more expertise in the pursuit of a very successful career in medical management. However, be forwarned that there will be some "sharks" in this pool. As always, your best defense is a good offense. That offense can best be developed from the many superb and readily available educational experiences offered through ACPE. Take advantage of these opportunities as frequently as possible. The rewards are immense.

The best of everything for a satisfying and successful new career.

Jerry L. Hammon, MD, FACPE
West Milton, Ohio
January 4, 1993

INDEX